DIARIES OF A MENTAL HEALTH NURSE

This book is a work of personal reflection based on the author's professional experiences in mental health nursing. Certain names, identifying details, locations, and circumstances may have been changed or adapted to protect privacy, confidentiality, and professional boundaries.

The views and experiences expressed in this book are those of the author. They are not intended to represent the views, policies, or practices of any specific healthcare organisation, employer, institution, or professional body.

This book is intended for general reading, reflection, and educational interest only. It should not be used as a substitute for professional medical, psychological, legal, or clinical advice.

Published by Cleo Raem

ISBN Paperback: 978-1-0666326-4-0

First Edition 1st 2026

Table of Contents

First Shift

I had never worked a 12-hour shift before. As a nursing student, I was always sent home early. My mentors would say, "You're only a student, one day you'll do the full shift."

That day had finally come.

I woke up early that morning, full of nervous energy but also excitement. This was it, my first shift as a fully qualified nurse. No longer a student. No longer observing. I was part of the team now.

Walking into the unit felt daunting. Everything suddenly seemed more real, more serious. The responsibility sat heavily, even before I had done a single task.

As I pulled up a chair to sit down, I could feel my legs shaking.

The ward manager was there and introduced me to everyone on the team. Faces blurred into one another as names were exchanged. I nodded, smiled, trying to take it all in while steadying the nerves bubbling underneath.

The night nurse began her handover. As she spoke, she looked directly at me. I couldn't tell if it was intentional or not, but it made me feel exposed, like all eyes were on me, waiting to see if I could handle it.

Still, I kept my composure. On the outside, I was calm. Inside, my mind was racing.

After the handover, the manager asked me to step into her office. She assigned me a preceptor, a senior nurse who would guide me through my first six months, and explained how the preceptorship would work. There was a book, a guide to everything expected of a nurse in charge, and I would work through it step by step, building up my confidence and competence along the way.

When I returned to the ward, I passed a group of the lads. They stopped me and asked who I was.

"I'm a new staff nurse," I said, the words still feeling unfamiliar in my mouth.

They introduced themselves, easy and welcoming, and told me that if I needed anything, they'd help me out. That moment stayed with me.

In the middle of all the uncertainty, it was a small but important reassurance, I wasn't alone.

We made our way to the clinic room to begin the day. My preceptor walked me through everything, what was stored where, how things were organised. Even though I was now a qualified nurse, she still went through it as if I were a student. I didn't mind... but I noticed it.

I collected the drug trolley and began the morning medication round. The patients were already lining up by the half-door, the kind where you can open the top and bottom separately. My preceptor stayed in the clinic room. I had my PIN, my personal registration number, the thing that makes a nurse legally responsible for every medication they give. I didn't need supervision anymore.

That hit me.

I was now responsible. I was now a qualified nurse.

There were fewer than ten patients on the unit, an assessment ward within a secure unit. As I went through the medications, I spoke with each patient. I asked them what they were taking. Some could tell me, others couldn't, so I explained it to them. Thankfully, I still remembered a lot of the psychiatric medications, there are so many, and it's easy to forget. When needed, I referred to the BNF, the British National Formulary, which is the reference book nurses and doctors use for medication information.

After the medication round, I returned to the office. My preceptor reassured me that she would work at my pace and support me whenever needed, but ultimately, the responsibility was mine. She asked how I wanted to structure my day.

"I just want to get on with it," I told her.

I even offered to do the evening handover, on my first day.

She smiled and said no.

I carried a small notebook in my pocket. Throughout the day, I jotted things down, conversations with patients, updates from staff, anything important. I reviewed patient files to understand their histories. This wasn't an easy ward. Many of the patients had been referred through the courts for assessment. The multidisciplinary team, doctors, nurses, psychologists, social workers, had to determine whether they were mentally fit to stand trial or required treatment instead.

These were not straightforward cases.

At one point, I was asked to complete a care plan for a recently admitted patient. I remember thinking to myself: A.P.I.E, Assessment, Planning, Implementation, Evaluation. Back to basics. Back to what we learned in training. I completed the care plan, and my preceptor reviewed it. She made a few small additions, but overall, she was happy with it.

I was relieved.

Sometime around midday, though the exact timing is a bit of a blur, the alarms went off.

Even though I had completed my training in the management of violence and aggression, I wasn't assigned as a responder. I was still supernumerary, there in a learning capacity, not yet counted in the staffing numbers. One of the nurses responded immediately. My preceptor turned to me and said, "If you want to go, you can, but you don't have to."

I went.

What I saw stayed with me.

I had never witnessed that level of aggression before. It took five members of staff to restrain one patient. As a student, you're often shielded from these situations. You're usually redirected, asked to support other patients, and to stay away from the incident itself.

But this time, I saw everything.

And it was overwhelming.

While watching the restraint, my thoughts weren't just about what was happening physically. I kept thinking about the patient. What must that feel like? To be confused, frightened, possibly paranoid, and suddenly held down by five people. To believe you're being attacked when, in reality, people are trying to keep you safe.

That thought stayed with me.

The restraint lasted several minutes, five, maybe a bit longer. Eventually, the patient calmed down. A healthcare assistant he trusted was able to talk him through it and guide him to a quieter area.

We returned to our ward.

I remember thinking, This is my first day.

Back on the unit, I spoke with my preceptor about what I had seen. We had a debrief, she gave me space to process it, to talk through how I felt. She explained that the unit I was working on could be particularly challenging. It was an assessment ward. Patients didn't want to be there. Emotions were heightened. Situations could escalate quickly.

I understood that.

Still, seeing it firsthand was something else.

By the end of the shift, I had given my handover on my first day.

I thanked the team. They had been incredibly supportive throughout. It hadn't been an easy introduction, but it had been real.

That evening, I went home and had a shower, almost like I was trying to wash the day off me. Then I sat down and, without even trying, started reflecting on everything that had happened.

Am I actually in the right job?

Did I choose the right setting? Secure services... was this really for me?

I told myself, " Look, give it a month. Just one month. Then decide.

At the back of my mind, I already had an interview lined up with another organisation. So I suppose I gave myself an option, a way out, just in case. But still, I made that decision: in one month, and I'll know.

That night, I journaled everything. Broke the day down bit by bit.

Even though I wasn't directly involved in the restraint, it stayed with me. I didn't have all the details, but I knew the staff involved had a post-incident debrief. I remember wishing I could have been there, to understand it more, to learn from it. Later, I reviewed the documentation. I think that was my way of trying to make sense of it all.

Looking back, that was really the moment I started journaling seriously. At the time, it wasn't about writing a "diary" like this, it was reflective practice. After each shift, especially the difficult ones, I'd sit down and ask myself:

How did the shift go? Could I have done anything differently? Was I happy with how I worked? Were my colleagues okay with how things went?

It became a habit without me even realising.

Now, having gone through different levels of management, all the way up to Head of Nursing, I can see how important that was. That simple act of reflecting after each shift shaped how I grew, how I learned, and how I support others now.

But back then, sitting there after my very first shift, all I really knew was this:

It made me think.

Day Two

I tossed and turned that night. But weirdly enough, the next morning I woke up feeling fully rested. Got washed, dressed, ready for work, hopped into my little car, and drove back.

As soon as I walked in, I didn't feel uneasy anymore. Felt like I belonged, strange, because it was only my second day.

Straight into handover. My preceptor was there. Once it finished, she turned to me, I still don't know why, and said, "Cleo". What do you want us to do? Where do you want us to go?"

So I led on my second day.

I went through the diary, allocated duties based on what was planned, and felt great. Weirdly relaxed. Did the medication round. Then had a meeting with the consultant psychiatrist about a new patient, referred by the courts for assessment. My preceptor and the full MDT: Forensic Consultant Psychiatrist, Consultant Psychologist, Occupational Therapist, and Social Worker.

The patient had been referred following a serious offence. We were asked to assess whether he was mentally stable enough to stand trial over the coming months.

Sitting there, I thought: This is me. I'm here, with all these highly intelligent professionals, and they want my opinion. Based on what was presented, I agreed that the person needed further assessment in our unit.

At the end of the day, the doctor confirmed we would accept the referral. My preceptor called me into the office afterwards and told me the consultant psychiatrist had assumed I was near the end of my preceptorship. She'd had no idea it was only my second day.

I felt happy and proud, not just because of the compliment, but because I felt at ease. The team had welcomed me so warmly on the first day that I could really open up on the second.

I'm naturally an open person, I suppose. So I just felt comfortable being myself.

Went home that day feeling absolutely great.

Day Three

By the third day, something had shifted.

The ward already felt familiar. Not in the way somewhere feels familiar after years, but in the way a rhythm does. I could sense the pace before the handover had even finished. I knew where things were. I knew which patients needed more time, which voices to watch for.

There was a small incident in the lounge mid-morning, a patient flared up, nothing serious. The staff member with the best rapport with him stepped in and led it. I moved the other patients away from the scene quietly and calmly.

Went home that evening tired, but in a different way. Not the exhaustion of overwhelm, more the tiredness of effort. Of being properly present for twelve hours.

I was starting to understand what the job actually felt like from the inside.

First Restraint

My first restraint as a fully qualified nurse happened in my second week.

Alarms went off. I'd been allocated as the first responder, so I ran to the adjacent unit. A patient had attacked and poured on a member of staff and was attempting to attack fellow peers. As I got there, without thinking, I went straight into the restaurant.

It all happened so fast. I took hold of the patient's left arm while another colleague took the right. It was almost in sync, like we'd rehearsed it. Using aggression management techniques, we worked together. The patient was so aggressive that we had to bring him to the ground. Two others took hold of his legs; another supported his head and took the lead in communicating. Only one person ever speaks during a restraint, and that's crucial. The patient was shouting, refusing to listen, but we held firm and followed what we had been taught.

Time seemed distorted. The person monitoring said it lasted ten minutes, but it felt like hours. Eventually, the patient agreed to follow the lead nurse to a quiet room. I expected refusal of medication, as I had seen that as a student. But surprisingly, the patient requested an IM injection, an intramuscular injection, given directly into the muscle for faster effect, and even specified which medication. After receiving it, he calmed down in his bedroom.

Returning to my own ward, I was still shaking. Holding a struggling person down is not easy. I journaled it all after the shift, breaking down what I had witnessed. It made me question the ethics of restraint, but I reminded myself. This patient had poured hot water on a colleague and was a danger to others. The restraint was necessary.

The debrief afterwards was invaluable. Unlike in some places I've worked, I was called back to the unit to discuss what had happened, what had escalated the situation, and what could have been done differently. The ward staff acknowledged that maybe earlier responses could have prevented it, but importantly, everyone was safe. The patient was checked by the on-call doctor. No physical harm.

This was a huge learning moment for me. I'm grateful for the experience and the debrief. Still, I'll never forget the fear, the adrenaline, the responsibility of restraining someone. When I close my eyes, I sometimes still see it, running toward the unit, holding someone down, the weight of that moment on everyone involved.

It's not easy.

And it's not something I take lightly, for the patient or for the staff.

My First Unsupervised Injection

I was in the clinic room alone when it came back to me.

Near the end of my nurse training, my last placement, a community setting, my preceptor sat me down and said:

"Think about the last three years. Anything you've avoided, anything you're not confident with, tell me now. Because soon, you'll be on your own."

And I knew straight away what it was.

Injections.

I used to avoid them when I could. I'd feel it in my hands, that slight shake as I drew up medication from a vial. Sometimes I'd even catch myself holding my breath without realising.

So she sent me to a depot clinic. During this regular session, patients came in from the community, one after another, from nine to five. For long-acting medication delivered by injection at scheduled intervals. Injection after injection. No avoiding it. No hiding. At the time, it felt like exposure therapy.

Now, standing in the clinic room as a qualified nurse, those memories came flooding back.

Except this time, there was no preceptor.

No one to check with.

No one to step in.

Just me.

I prepared the injection. Checked it. Checked it again and asked a second nurse to check it

Trying to ignore that familiar feeling creeping back into my hands.

The patient came in.

I didn't rush it. Didn't overthink it either.

I just did it.

And afterwards, there was this quiet moment, nothing dramatic, nothing outwardly different.

But inside, I felt it.

Pride.

Because this time, I hadn't done it as a student. I hadn't done it with someone watching over me.

I'd done it alone.

And I realised… maybe I wasn't as unprepared as I thought.

***

A few months later, I had to do it again.

But this time… it was different.

There had been an incident on the unit. A patient had to be restrained. We tried everything first, talking, de-escalating, giving space where we could. But nothing was working.

I was told to go and prepare the IM medication.

I rushed to the clinic room.

Two injections.

As I was drawing up the medication, my hands were shaking, properly shaking this time. Not like before. This felt different. More pressure. More urgency.

But there was no time to stand there thinking about it.

I checked the doses. Checked for bubbles. Tried to steady my hands.

Then I went back.

The restraint was still ongoing. The atmosphere was tense, controlled, but tense. My colleagues repositioned the patient so I could access the injection site. Everything felt fast, but also slowed down at the same time.

I remember thinking: Don't get this wrong.

I administered the injection into the outer upper quadrant of the buttock while the patient was still fighting.

I could feel myself shivering.

Not just nerves, fear.

Fear that I might hurt them.

Fear that I might do something wrong.

Fear of the responsibility sitting entirely on me in that moment.

But I did it.

And then… we waited.

Gradually, the medication began to take effect. The patient settled. The fight eased. Eventually, we were able to talk, really talk, about what had led up to everything.

Afterwards, we had a debrief. I spoke about how it felt, doing that for the first time in a restraint, in that kind of situation. How difficult it was to stay focused when everything in you is heightened. The team was supportive. They understood.

Then came the paperwork. The incident forms. The documentation. Informing the right people. The patient was reviewed by the doctor and physically checked over. Observations were conducted regularly to ensure safety and no complications.

Because that's the other side of it.

You don't just give the medication and walk away.

You carry the responsibility for what happens after.

And that stayed with me, not just that I did it, but everything that came with it.

When You Have to Say No

Working 12-hour shifts, you really get to know your patients.

You notice the small changes. The patterns. The way someone reacts to certain words, certain tones, and certain situations. You build a rapport that doesn't come from a quick assessment; it comes from time.

I remember one particular shift.

There was a patient who had been unsettled. Not aggressive, just very psychotic. We knew him. We'd seen these phases before. We knew how he presented.

He wasn't a danger.

But during an MDT discussion, a meeting with the full multidisciplinary team, one of the doctors was adamant that he needed to be secluded.

Seclusion.

Locked in a room. Alone.

To us, that was a last resort, something you use when someone is actively aggressive, when there is no other safe option left.

This wasn't that.

The nursing team, including me, pushed back. We explained that he wasn't aggressive. That he could be managed. That he needed support, observation, and probably medication, not isolation.

But the doctor stood firm.

There was this unspoken expectation, I'm the doctor, so this is the decision.

I remember feeling it clearly.

And I remember saying no.

I was the nurse in charge that shift. And I wasn't going to authorise isolating someone who wasn't a danger to anyone.

It didn't go down well.

A meeting followed. We were reported. I reported myself to the ward manager straight away. When she came to speak to me, she agreed there was no justification for seclusion in this case.

But it didn't end there.

It was escalated to the Director of Nursing. The next day, myself and the ward manager were called in. We explained everything, our reasoning, our knowledge of the patient, and the context.

And the Director of Nursing agreed with us.

Because we knew that patient. We had spent twelve hours with him. The doctor had seen him for minutes.

And that mattered.

The patient was never secluded. He remained on the ward, supported, observed. And the phase passed. No harm came to anyone.

About a week later, before a ward round, the doctor approached me.

"I hope there's no hard feelings," he said.

And there wasn't.

Because this isn't about being right or wrong. It's about the patient. I told him exactly that, we both did what we thought was best, and that was enough. I appreciated that he had come to me.

You can't hold grudges in this job. Not in an environment where you rely on each other. Where things can change in seconds.

So we moved on.

The patient stayed safe.

No one was harmed.

And that's what mattered.

I remember writing about it afterwards, thinking, sometimes the hardest part of this job isn't the patients.

It's having the confidence to speak up for them.

The ‘Tricky’ Area

One of the biggest things you don't fully understand until you're in the job is how often care and control sit side by side.

When you come into mental health nursing, you think your role is to help, to support, to listen. And it is. But there's another side to it that people don't really talk about enough, the side where you have to override someone's wishes for what you believe is the right reason.

Medication is where this hits hardest.

Antipsychotics, mood stabilisers, rapid tranquillisers, you see them used in all sorts of ways. And most of the time, patients take them willingly. Maybe not happily, but they take them.

But then there are the times when they don't.

And that's when everything changes.

You can have someone in front of you who is clearly unwell, psychotic, distressed, not sleeping, not eating properly, maybe paranoid, maybe hearing voices, and they are telling you, clearly, repeatedly, "I don't want medication."

And you stand there knowing that medication could help them. That it might bring them back to themselves. That, without it, they might deteriorate further.

But they're still saying no.

That's the ‘tricky’ area.

Because in any other setting in healthcare, a patient refusing treatment is often the end of the conversation. But in mental health, under the Mental Health Act, it's not always that simple.

The decision moves beyond just the patient. It becomes about risk, capacity, and safety, both theirs and others'.

And sometimes, the decision is made that medication will be given regardless of consent.

I remember that early in my career, it was something I really struggled with.

Not the theory of it, I understood the reasoning. But the reality of it is very different.

It's one thing to say someone needs medication.

It's another thing entirely to be part of the team that has to give it when they're actively refusing.

Because it doesn't just mean handing over tablets.

Sometimes it means restraint. Alarms are going off. Staff running from different parts of the ward. That shift in atmosphere where everything suddenly becomes focused, intense. You already know, before you even arrive, that it's not going to be a calm conversation.

And then you're there, hands on a patient, holding them, not out of anger, not out of punishment, but because that's what the situation has come to.

And in that moment, they're not seeing care.

They're seeing control.

They're seeing people holding them down, taking away their choice, and injecting them with something they've already said they don't want.

That's not something you brush off.

I remember after some of those early incidents, going home and replaying it in my head. Thinking about what the patient must have felt like. Questioning whether it was right, even when I knew, clinically and legally, it was justified.

You carry that with you in the beginning.

Over time, something shifts.

You start to see the outcomes. You see patients who were once completely overwhelmed by their illness begin to settle. You see them sleep again. Eat again. Talk more clearly. Sometimes, you even hear them say later on that the medication helped.

And that changes your perspective.

It doesn't make it easy, but it gives it context.

You begin to understand that, in mental health, sometimes doing the right thing doesn't always look or feel like the right thing in the moment. It can feel uncomfortable. It can feel intrusive. It can feel like you're crossing a line.

But you also start to understand that if you didn't act, if you stood back and did nothing in the name of autonomy, the outcome could be far worse.

That doesn't mean you stop thinking about it.

Even now, when those situations come up, I still pause internally. There's always that moment of awareness, of what's about to happen, of what it means.

And I think that's important.

Because the day you stop thinking about it completely, the day it becomes routine or mechanical, that's when you lose something essential in this job.

This role isn't just about following procedures or administering medication.

It's about holding that balance between care and control, constantly.

And accepting that sometimes, you'll be standing right in the middle of that 'tricky' area, knowing there isn't a perfect answer, just the best decision you can make in that moment.

All you can do is act with care, with thought, with respect for the person in front of you. And hope that, in the end, it helps them find some stability, some peace.

That's what keeps me in this work, even on the hardest days.

A 12-Hour Shift

Someone messaged me recently. She wasn't in healthcare, wasn't a nurse, but she said she always heard about twelve-hour shifts and how long they were, and she wanted to know, what do nurses actually do for those twelve hours?

I thought about it. Unless you've worked one, you don't really see it. So this is what a shift looks like.

***

Seven fifteen. I always try to get in a bit early, not because I have to, but because I need those few minutes to settle myself before the day starts. You never really know what you're walking into.

By half past seven, we're all gathered for handover. The night nurse goes through each patient. Who slept. Who didn't? Who was up all night pacing. Who needed something extra? Any incidents, any concerns. Sometimes it's quiet. Sometimes you hear things that make you sit up a bit straighter, building a picture in your head before you've even stepped onto the ward properly.

Handover can take fifteen minutes, sometimes thirty. It depends on the night.

Once that's done, the shift really begins. If I'm the nurse in charge, I grab the diary straight away. Appointments, hospital runs, reviews, therapy sessions. You scan through it quickly but properly, because missing something small can turn into a big problem later.

Then comes allocation. Who's doing medications, who's on observations, and who's the responder if alarms go off? Patient allocations get split between the staff, and the morning starts to move.

Medications go out first thing. Some patients are up and waiting, some you have to wake. While that's happening, the rest of the ward is moving, breakfast, checks, and conversations are starting. You're scanning constantly. Body language. Tone. Who's withdrawn this morning who wasn't yesterday? Whose pacing? Who hasn't said a word?

Mid-morning is when meetings tend to happen. Multidisciplinary review, doctors, psychologists, occupational therapists, social workers, all in one room, going through patients one by one. Risks. Plans.

Progress. Discharges, transfers, leave applications. As the nurse, you're often the voice in the room with the most up-to-date picture of how someone actually is, because you've been with them. You feed that in. You raise concerns. You push when you need to.

Between meetings, you're back on the floor. Observations need writing up. Care plans need updating. A family has called and wants a return call. Somebody needs a one-to-one. Somebody else has had a difficult morning and needs space, or needs you to sit with them, or needs you to know it's not personal.

Lunch is rarely a break. You eat when you can. Sometimes you don't.

Afternoons run differently from mornings, but the rhythm is the same, scanning, responding, documenting, responding again. There are good afternoons where a patient who hasn't engaged in weeks sits down to talk, and there are afternoons where the alarms don't stop. You don't always get to choose which one you're walking into.

By late afternoon, you're preparing for the next handover and going back through the day. What happened, what didn't, what the night team needs to watch for. You write it all down because the next nurse has to be able to pick it up cleanly. That handover is somebody else's first impression of how the day went, and it's also the safety net for whoever comes next.

Half seven in the evening, twelve hours later, you walk out. Or that's the plan. Some shifts, you walk out at eight or half eight because something happened in the last half hour, and you couldn't leave it. You hand the keys over. You sign out.

And then you go home. But not really. Because mentally, sometimes you're still there. Running through the day and thinking about patients and wondering if everyone's okay.

People see twelve hours and think it's just time. It's not. It's constant thinking, constant observing, constant responsibility. And no two shifts are ever the same.

A 12-Hour Night Shift

After explaining what a day shift looks like, I thought I might as well talk about nights, too. Because people hear "night shift" and assume it's quiet. That nothing really happens. Once everyone is asleep, that's it.

It's not like that.

The night shift still starts the same way. Twelve hours. The night staff come in and take handover from the day team, what's happened, who's been unsettled, who's at risk, who needs close monitoring. You pick up the shift where the day staff left off, but the energy is different. The ward starts to slow down. It doesn't switch off.

Earlier in the evening, there are still activities on offer, but they're different. More relaxed. Less structured. Nothing too heavy, because the aim is to start helping people wind down. Some patients watch television. Some sit and talk with the staff. Some just want quiet. There's no big group meeting like during the day; it's more individual, more flexible. You go at the patient's pace.

And then, slowly, the ward begins to settle. Or that's the aim.

One of the biggest priorities on a night shift is sleep. People underestimate how important sleep is in mental health. If someone doesn't sleep properly, it affects everything, their mood, their thinking, and their ability to engage the next day. So a big part of the role at night is promoting sleep, encouraging routines, and offering support. Medication if needed.

But it's not always straightforward. Not everyone sleeps. There are always patients who are awake, some pacing, some anxious, some unable to switch off. And sometimes the night is when people open up. You'll sit with someone at two in the morning, and they'll start telling you how they really feel. Things they didn't say during the day. Things they've been holding in. In those moments, you're not just there to observe. You're there to listen, to support, to hold the space.

While all of that is happening, there's another side to night shifts that people don't see, the behind-the-scenes work. This is when a lot of the housekeeping gets done. Going through documentation. Making sure everything is filed properly. Checking standards are being maintained. Reviewing care plans. Updating assessments. Checking the clinic room. Making sure everything is in order for the next day. It's quiet work, but it matters. If things aren't right behind the scenes, it shows during the day.

Just because it's night doesn't mean it's calm. You can still have patients become distressed, incidents occur, and alarms go off. You still need to respond quickly, safely, and professionally. There's no "it's night, so it's easier." Sometimes it's harder, fewer staff, less immediate backup. You rely on each other more.

And then there are the checks. Regular observations throughout the night. Walking quietly through the ward, trying not to wake anyone, making sure people are breathing, settled, okay. Always alert. Always aware.

People often say, "Night shift must be handy, everyone's asleep." But they're not. Or at least, not all of them. And even when they are, you're still working and still thinking. Still responsible. Still carrying the ward through until morning.

Before you know it, it's the early hours. Then five. Then six. The ward slowly begins to wake up again. You begin preparing for handover, what's happened overnight, who struggled, who didn't sleep, who needs reviewing. You pass it on to the day staff, just like it was passed to you.

And just like that, another twelve hours are done. Night shifts are different. Quieter, but not easy. Slower, but still demanding. A different kind of nursing, but still nursing. Still care—still responsibility. Still work.

"Are Patients Just Locked Up All Day?"

Someone asked me this once. They weren't being rude; they were genuinely curious. "When people are in the hospital," they said, "are they just locked up all day? Like, do they ever get to go out?"

A lot of people probably think that. Once someone is admitted, that's it. Four walls. No freedom. No normal life.

It's not like that. Yes, it's a hospital. Yes, there are restrictions. But people don't just get locked away and forgotten about. They still have rights. And part of our job as nurses is to balance those rights with safety, for the patient and for the public.

When it comes to going out into the community, there's no one-size-fits-all approach. Everything is based on assessment. What setting are you in, acute, rehab, or forensic? What is the patient's current mental state? What are the risks? Can they go out alone, or do they need support?

Some patients can go out independently. Others need staff with them. And that support isn't always about risk. Sometimes it's because someone is anxious, hasn't been out in a while, or has lost confidence. So you go with them, not to watch them, but to support them. Other times, their mental health doesn't allow them to be out alone yet safely. That's okay too.

In most settings, activities are planned with the nursing and occupational therapy teams. They look at what's available in the community, meaningful things, enjoyable things, things that help people rebuild a sense of normal life. Because that's what it's about. Normality.

I remember one day in particular. We took a group of patients to the beach. It was something they had been talking about for a while, something simple, but important to them. So we planned it properly. Risk-assessed it. Organised transport. Made sure everyone was safe. And we went.

Honestly, it was one of those days that remind you why you do the job. Just being out. Fresh air. People laughing. Talking. For a moment, it didn't feel like a hospital. It just felt normal.

That's the thing: people don't always realise that we're not just treating symptoms. We're helping people reconnect with life. Some patients like going to the library. Some want to go shopping, pick out their own food, and cook their own meals. Some just want a coffee somewhere that isn't a hospital.

I've been asked, "Would you ever take a patient to the pub?" The answer is yes. I've worked in places where we've gone to the pub. Not for alcohol, but for a meal, a drink, a bit of normal social interaction. Because when someone is discharged, they're going back into the real world. And part of our role is helping them prepare for that.

I've taken patients to concerts. I've supported people on short trips away, even overnight stays, depending on the setting and what's been agreed. Every place is different. Every patient is different. But the principle stays the same.

People are not in the hospital to be punished. They're there to be supported. So no, patients are not locked up all day. They do go out. They do engage in the community. They do normal things. But everything is done with purpose, with planning, with safety in mind because it's about helping someone get back to a place where they can live their life again. Not just exist within four walls.

Inspections

Inspections are part of the job, whether people realise it or not.

As nurses, we don't just care for patients. We're also part of preparing for inspections. The regulatory body changes depending on where you work, but when the inspectors arrive, they come to the nurses first. We're on the frontline. We know the patients. We know the systems. So naturally, we're the ones being asked the questions.

They speak to the wider team, doctors, occupational therapists, and management. Still, a lot of it comes back to us, about what we're doing day to day, how we're documenting, how we're keeping patients safe. Because that's what inspections are really about. Safety, standards, accountability. Making sure we're doing what we say we're doing.

I remember my first inspection. I was properly nervous. The kind where your hands feel shaky, and your mind goes blank, even though you know your job. At the time, it felt like someone was coming in to question everything I was doing. Am I doing this right? What if I miss something? What if I can't answer?

It wasn't like that. The inspector I spoke to could see straight away that I was nervous. He paused and said, "I can see you're a bit anxious, that's okay." Then he explained why he was there. Not to catch me out. Not to criticise for the sake of it. But to ensure standards were being met and to help improve things if needed. That changed everything for me.

He asked me to show him a care plan. Simple enough, but in that moment, it didn't feel simple. Then he asked about audits. Back then, I wasn't heavily involved in auditing. I was honest about that. I said no, but I could show him where the audit schedule was, who was responsible, and how it was organised.

That mattered. It's not about knowing everything. It's about being safe, honest, and aware.

They look at everything. Care plans. Risk assessments. Training records. Audits. Documentation. Patient involvement. It's detailed, but it has to be. Because if you look back at the history of mental health services, before bodies like these existed, standards weren't always good. There were safeguarding failures. There was neglect. There was abuse. And that's the part people sometimes forget.

Inspections aren't just about checking on patients; they're about protecting them. But they're also there to protect us. Because when you're documenting properly, following guidelines, and evidencing your practice, you're safeguarding your own registration too.

Over the years, I've been through many inspections. That nervous feeling never fully goes away, but it changes. You start to understand what they're looking for. You learn how to prepare. You help others prepare. You become the calm one in the room instead of the anxious one.

Now I see inspections for what they are. Necessary. Important. Protective. Even if they do make your heart race a little when they first walk onto the ward.

Owning Up

Owning up to mistakes. It sounds simple, but it's one of the hardest things to do in this job.

Over the years, I've seen how difficult it is for people. To be fair, there's a reason for that. People are scared. Scared of losing their job. Scared of being labelled incompetent. Scared of being judged.

But the truth is, mistakes happen. And in nursing, when they happen, they can put patients or colleagues at risk. That's why owning up matters.

I remember one incident clearly. I was administering a controlled drug. As nurses, we know the rule: controlled drugs require two signatures. Two nurses are present. No shortcuts. But that day, I gave the medication without getting the second signature. I remember thinking, I'll get it after.

That's not how it works. It should be done there and then. Properly. Safely. By the book. Because the moment you don't, you create a risk. And in this case, it led to a discrepancy.

I had a choice. Say nothing, or speak up. I spoke up. I said, "That was me. I didn't get the second signature." And that was it. There was no shouting. No humiliation. Just a conversation. I was told clearly, " Don't let it happen again. And more importantly, why it should never happen again.

That stayed with me.

It wasn't the only mistake I've made. I've given the wrong medication before. Similar names. Similar packaging. Busy medication round. Patients waiting, queuing, asking, "Can I have mine now?" No excuse. I should have slowed down. But I didn't. And I picked up the wrong box.

Again, I had a choice. Ignore it, or report it. I followed the procedure. Incident form completed. Team informed. Patient reviewed. Thankfully, no harm was done. But that wasn't the point. The point was this: if you don't own up, you don't learn properly. You might tell yourself you'll do better next time, but it's different when you actually face it, acknowledge it, and reflect on it. It makes you more aware. More careful. More accountable.

Now, when things get busy, when there's a queue, when there's pressure, I stop. I tell patients to wait. I ask for quiet. I take control of the situation because rushing is where mistakes happen. And medication errors are not something you ever want to take lightly.

Owning up doesn't make you a bad nurse. Hiding mistakes does. Owning up makes you safer. It protects your patients, and it protects you.

You won't ever go through your career without making a mistake. But you can decide what kind of nurse you'll be when it happens.

***

In nursing, accountability isn't optional; it's a professional duty. The regulatory bodies are clear on it: nurses must practise safely, be open and honest, and raise concerns when things go wrong. The word for it is professional candour.

Owning up to mistakes isn't just good practice; it's essential. It's part of maintaining your registration. Failing to disclose an error, especially one that could affect patient safety, has serious legal and professional consequences. But when you are honest, when you follow policy, when you report and reflect, you demonstrate insight. And insight matters. It shows you are safe to practise. It shows you are willing to learn. It shows you are accountable.

What I've learned is this: slow down, no matter how busy it gets. Never take shortcuts with medication. Follow policy, especially when under pressure. Speak up immediately when something goes wrong. Create an environment where it's safe for others to admit mistakes. And learn from every error, don't bury it.

Team Building

Team building. It sounds like one of those buzzwords people throw around in meetings, but in nursing, it's real. And it matters.

In my experience, over twenty years in nursing, team building is one of the most important parts of the job. Because we don't just work together. We spend long hours together. Twelve-hour shifts. Back-to-back days. High-pressure situations. You're not just colleagues. You become a unit.

That doesn't happen overnight. It takes time. The same way you build rapport with a patient who's just been admitted, slowly, consistently, with effort, it's the same with a team. New staff come in. Different personalities. Different ways of working. At first, it can feel a bit disconnected. But over time, you start to gel.

I've been part of different team-building activities over the years. Some simple, some more organised. Going for meals together, walking, or hiking. Even just spending time together outside the ward environment. Nothing complicated, but it makes a difference. You start to see people as more than just their role.

Something interesting happens when a team really knows each other. Communication becomes easier, not just what's said, but what's understood. You start to anticipate things. You know how your colleague thinks. You know how your doctor is likely to respond. You know when something will be approved, and when it won't.

A patient might say, "I want to stop my medication." If you know your team, especially your doctor, you already have a sense of what that conversation will look like. You're not guessing. You're aligned. The same applies across the board if a family member calls. Suppose another professional asks for information if decisions need to be made quickly. When the team knows each other, things flow. You don't have to second-guess everything.

In mental health settings, especially, that flow matters. Because when things don't flow, when communication breaks down, you feel it immediately. The shift becomes harder. Tension builds. Mistakes are more likely. You can always tell when a team isn't quite working. There's a disconnect. Someone feels off. Someone isn't communicating. Someone doesn't trust the process. And it affects everything.

But when does a team work? It's different. There's an unspoken understanding. Meetings run more smoothly. Decisions feel clearer. Support feels natural. Sometimes you don't even need to say much. People just get it.

Team building isn't about ticking a box. It's about creating an environment where people understand each other, communication is easier, trust is built, and the work feels manageable. Because no matter how experienced you are, you don't do this job alone. When the team works well, everything else follows.

I'll say this too. I've been lucky. Over the years, I've worked in some really good teams. I can honestly put my hand up and say I've worked with good people. People who supported each other. People who communicated. People who made difficult shifts feel that they were manageable. And when you've experienced that, you realise just how important a good team really is because not everyone gets that.

Confidentiality

Confidentiality. It's one of those things that sits quietly in the background of nursing, but it's constant. Always there. Always guiding what you say, and what you don't say.

A lot happens behind closed doors in mental health units, not in a negative way, but in a private, protected way. Patients share things. You witness things. You're trusted with things. And that trust has to be protected.

One thing people don't always realise is how careful you have to be outside of work. With family. With friends. In everyday conversations. People are naturally curious, especially when they know you work in mental health, and even more so in areas like forensic services. They'll ask things like, "What are your patients like?" "What did they do to end up there?" "Tell me something interesting that happened."

Most of the time, they don't mean any harm. They're just interested. They care about you. They want to understand your day. But our job isn't something we can openly talk about, not in detail. Not in the way people might expect.

I've had moments where people have tried to dig a little deeper. Nothing malicious, just curiosity. But that's where you have to draw a line. You have to be able to say, "I can't talk about that. It's confidential." And leave it there.

Over time, I've learned to keep things simple. "How was work?" "It was busy." "It was fine." "Long day." That's enough. Because once you share something, you lose control of it. Even if you trust the person you're telling, they might repeat it. Mention it casually. Tell someone else without thinking. "My friend told me about a patient who…", and just like that, something private becomes public.

Confidentiality isn't just about obvious details like names. It's everything. Situations. Circumstances. Stories. Anything that could identify a patient, directly or indirectly. And it's not just about rules. It's about respect. Patients come into our care at some of their most vulnerable moments. They trust that what happens in that environment stays there.

***

Confidentiality is a core part of professional practice. The regulatory guidance is clear: nurses must respect and protect patient information at all times, in and out of the workplace, in person, on the phone, and on social media. Breaching it, even unintentionally, has serious consequences. Not just professionally, but for the patient involved.

What I've learned is that not everyone needs to know what happens at work. Curiosity from others doesn't override confidentiality. Keep answers simple. Never share identifiable patient information, even casually. Once information is shared, you lose control of it. Confidentiality is about trust, not just policy.

It isn't just a rule we follow. It's a responsibility we carry every single day.

Boundaries, When Caring Doesn't Mean Sharing

Boundaries. You learn them over time in nursing, not always from books, but from experience.

Because caring comes naturally, you want to help. You want to listen. You want to be there for people. But caring doesn't mean giving everything of yourself.

In mental health nursing, the relationships you build with patients can be strong. You spend long hours together. You see people at their most vulnerable. You support them through difficult moments. And because of that, boundaries can sometimes blur.

Patients might ask personal questions. "Do you have children?" "Where do you live?" "Are you married?" At first, it can feel harmless, and sometimes you might answer small things without thinking. But you have to be careful. Once you start sharing, it can be hard to pull it back.

Over the years, I've learned that it's okay to be warm without being personal. You can be kind. You can be supportive. You can build rapport. Without giving away parts of your private life. It's not about being cold. It's about being professional.

There have been times when patients have tried to get closer, not in a harmful way, but in a human way. They want a connection. They want familiarity. And sometimes, they test those boundaries. You might hear, "You're my favourite nurse," or "You understand me more than the others." That can feel nice to hear, but it's something you have to manage carefully. The relationship has to stay therapeutic, not personal.

Boundaries also protect you. They stop emotional burnout. They stop over-involvement. They keep things safe for both sides. Over time, you learn how to redirect conversations. How to gently bring the patient back. How to say no without making someone feel rejected. It's a skill. And like everything else in nursing, it takes practice.

When Patients Recognise You Outside the Ward

This is something people don't really prepare you for, seeing patients outside of work. It can catch you off guard.

You're in the shop. Out with family. Walking down the street. And suddenly, you see them. Or they see you.

I remember the first time it happened to me. I wasn't in uniform. I was just going about my day. And then I heard my name. I turned around, and it was a patient.

In that moment, you don't always know what to do. Do you acknowledge them? Do you keep walking? Do you speak? Because confidentiality comes into it again. You're now in a public space. Other people are around. And you have to think not just about yourself, but about them. What if they're with family who don't know they're under mental health services? What if someone overhears?

Over time, I've learned to take my lead from the patient. If they acknowledge me, I respond politely and briefly. If they don't, I respect that. You keep it neutral. A simple hello. A quick exchange. Nothing more. You don't start conversations about the ward. You don't mention anything clinical. You don't blur that line.

It can feel strange at first. Because you know them in one setting, and suddenly you're seeing them in another. But you have to remember that, outside the ward, they are just people living their lives. And you are too.

Knowing When to Switch Off

Knowing when to switch off, that's one I still struggle with.

The truth is, we care. You don't come into this profession if you don't. No one signs up to work in mental health, to support people at their most vulnerable, and then just walks away unaffected. It doesn't work like that.

Some moments stay with you. Things you've seen. Things you've heard. Situations that don't sit right. And sometimes they follow you home. That's where switching off becomes difficult. Because even when you leave the ward, your mind doesn't always leave with you.

There have been times when people close to me have noticed it. "You don't seem yourself." "Something's on your mind." And they're right. But you can't just open up and explain everything. Confidentiality still applies. So you carry it quietly.

That's why support is so important. Over the years, I've learned that you can't do this job alone. You need people. Whether that's supervision, reflective practice, workplace support services, or simply a trusted colleague. In every place I've worked, I've always found one or two people I can go to. People I trust. People I can speak to openly, within professional boundaries.

When I do, it helps. Because sometimes, when you're in the middle of a situation, you can't see it clearly. You're too involved. Too close to it. But when you speak to someone else, they help you step back. They break it down. They might say, "Look at it from this angle." "You did this right." "Maybe next time, try it this way." Not because you're incapable of reflecting on yourself, but because sometimes you need another perspective. We all do.

I've done the same for others. Sat down with colleagues. Talked things through. Helped them see situations more clearly. That's part of being a team.

Because if you don't switch off, it catches up with you. I've seen it happen. People are becoming overwhelmed. Burnt out. Taking work home every single day. And in some cases, it affects their personal lives. Relationships suffer. Energy drops. Everything starts to revolve around work.

That's where balance comes in. Work-life balance. We hear it all the time, especially from management or HR. But actually achieving it? That's the challenge. Because what works for one person won't work for another. You have to figure out what works for you. And sometimes that means saying no. No to extra shifts. No to overtime. No to things that will push you beyond your limit.

That's not always easy, especially when people pick up extra hours for financial reasons or personal commitments. I've done it myself. But as you go on, you start to recognise your limits. I know now, I can't do what I used to. And that's okay.

It's also important to recognise it in others. If you know your team well, you can see when someone is tired. When they're drained. When they're doing too much. Sometimes just pointing it out can make a difference. Because not everyone realises they're burning out until it's too late.

Switching off isn't about not caring. It's about caring enough to protect yourself, too.

Burnout, When You've Given Too Much

Burnout doesn't happen overnight. It creeps in. At first, you don't notice it. You're just tired. A bit drained after shifts. Needing more rest than usual. You tell yourself it's normal. "It's just been a busy week."

But then the feeling doesn't go away. It lingers. You start to feel different at work. Things that didn't bother you before start to get to you. Small things feel big. Patience becomes shorter. You feel emotionally exhausted.

And the hardest part to admit is this: you don't feel like yourself anymore. In a caring profession, that's difficult. Because you're used to being the one who supports others. The one who listens. The one who helps. But when you're burnt out, you start running on empty.

I've seen it in colleagues. Good nurses. Experienced nurses. People who gave everything to the job. And slowly, it took its toll. They stayed late. Picked up extra shifts. Carried more than they should have. Not because they had to, but because they cared. That's the thing about burnout. It often comes from caring too much, for too long, without enough support.

Sometimes it shows up physically. Constant fatigue. Trouble sleeping. Feeling run down. Sometimes it's emotional. Feeling detached. Irritable. Overwhelmed. And sometimes you don't even realise it's happening until someone else points it out. "You don't seem yourself." "You look exhausted."

That's why knowing your team matters. Your colleagues will often see it before you do. And when it's recognised early, it can be managed. If it's ignored, it builds.

I've learned that burnout isn't something to push through. It's something to address. That might mean taking time off. Reducing hours. Speaking to someone. Accessing support services. It might mean having difficult conversations. Saying, "I'm not okay." "I need a break." That's not easy, especially in a profession where you're used to being strong for others.

But the reality is this: if you don't look after yourself, you can't properly look after anyone else. I've also seen what happens when burnout isn't addressed. People leave the profession. People lose their passion. People struggle in their personal lives. And that's something we don't talk about enough.

Burnout doesn't mean you're weak. It means you've been strong for too long, without enough support.

A Wake-Up Call

In line with burnout, I'll share something personal.

I had a mini stroke. Something I never expected. It came as a shock.

Because when you think of strokes, you think of certain risk factors. High blood pressure. Underlying health conditions. A certain age group. I didn't fit that picture. My vitals were fine. No known issues. Nothing that would have made me think, this could happen to me.

But it did. And even now, I still question it. Was it stress? Was it something underlying? Was it just one of those things? I don't have all the answers.

What I do know is this: it made me stop. It made me reflect. On my health. On my lifestyle. On how much I give to this job. I don't even do excessive overtime. I've learned my limits over the years. And still, something like that happened.

So it makes you think. Maybe it was just a random event. Or maybe it was a sign. To slow down. To pay attention. To look after myself properly. Because in this job, it's easy to focus on everyone else, patients, colleagues, the ward, and somewhere along the way, you can forget about yourself.

That experience reminded me that anything can happen. At any time. Even when you think you're doing everything right. So now, more than ever, I take it seriously. Rest. Balance. Listening to my body. Because no job, no matter how important, is worth your health.

If you're not well, you can't care for anyone else. Sometimes it takes something unexpected to make you stop and reassess. For me, that was my wake-up call. And if there's one thing I've taken from it, it's this: don't wait for something to happen before you start looking after yourself.

Why I Stayed

After everything, the long shifts, the pressure, the responsibility, the moments that stay with you, the mistakes, the lessons, the burnout, even the health scare, why did I stay?

It's a question people have asked me over the years. "How do you do it?" "Why don't you leave?" "Is it really worth it?" There were times I asked myself the same thing. Days, I went home exhausted. Days I questioned if I was in the right job. Moments where things didn't feel fair. Moments where the system felt heavy.

But even in all of that, there was always something that kept me here. The patients. Not every day is a breakthrough. Not every story has a perfect ending. But there are moments, small moments that stay with you. A patient who was once withdrawn is starting to engage. Someone who couldn't trust is beginning to open up. A simple thank you from someone who's been through so much. Those moments matter. More than people realise.

And then there's the team. The people you work alongside. The ones who understand the job without you having to explain it. The ones who support you on the hard days.

The ones who make you laugh in the middle of chaos. That sense of not being alone, it matters.

Over time, this job becomes more than just a job. It becomes part of who you are. You grow in it. You learn. You adapt. You become stronger, not just clinically, but emotionally.

You start to see things differently. You understand people differently. You develop patience, empathy, and resilience.

Even on the hardest days, there's a sense that what you're doing matters. It's not always visible. It's not always recognised. But it matters.

I stayed because of that. Because even though the job can be tough, it's also meaningful. Because even though it can drain you, it can also fulfil you. And because deep down, I know I make a difference. Not every day. Not in every situation. But enough. Enough to stay.

Staying in a demanding profession like mental health nursing isn't just about endurance. It's about purpose. Purpose can carry you through difficult times. Small moments can have a big impact. Support from colleagues makes a difference. Growth comes through experience, both good and bad. Not every day will feel rewarding, and that's okay. Making a difference doesn't always look obvious. Sometimes, enough is enough reason to stay.

Training and Development

Training can sometimes feel like a tick-box exercise. But it's far more than that. Whether it's mandatory training or professional development, it matters.

We all have the basics we have to complete. Mandatory training. The things you have to stay up to date with. Yes, sometimes it can feel repetitive. But it's there for a reason. To keep patients safe. To keep us safe. To keep standards consistent.

Beyond that, there's professional development, and that's where the responsibility shifts a little onto us. Because things change. They change fast. I remember when I first trained. We used to learn care planning in a very structured way, assessment, planning, implementation, and evaluation, almost like a formula. Back then, it worked. But when you look at care plans now, they've evolved. They're more detailed. More person-centred. More reflective of individual needs. If you don't keep up, you fall behind.

Not everything can be provided by the organisation. That's just reality. Budgets. Time. Resources. They can't fund every course or every opportunity. But that doesn't mean development stops. Over the years, I've found there's a lot out there. Free resources. Online courses. Webinars. Learning platforms through health and social care bodies. You just have to look. And be willing.

Professional development isn't just about ticking a box for your registration. It's about staying competent. Staying confident. Staying relevant in your practice. Especially for those early in their careers. If you want to progress, if you're thinking about promotions, specialist roles, or leadership, you have to invest in yourself. No one else can do that for you.

The more you learn, the more it reflects in your work. Your confidence grows. Your knowledge deepens. Your decision-making improves. It also makes the job easier. Because you understand more. You recognise patterns quicker. You feel more equipped to handle situations.

Training isn't just something you attend. It's something you carry into your practice every day.

From Student to Nurse, What They Don't Teach You

Becoming a nurse, you think you're ready. You've done the training. Passed the exams. Completed your placements. You've worked hard to get there.

Then your first shift comes, and reality hits. Because no matter how much you've learned, there are things you're just not taught.

You're not taught what it feels like to be fully responsible. To have your own registration. To sign medications. To make decisions that actually carry weight. As a student, there's always someone there, a safety net. A mentor. A supervisor. As a qualified nurse, that changes.

I remember that feeling clearly. That moment of realisation: It's on me now.

You're not taught how heavy that responsibility can feel, or how quickly you have to adapt. You're not taught how to manage everything at once, patients, documentation, phone calls, families, colleagues, all happening at the same time. It can feel overwhelming.

Then there's confidence. Or lack of it. You might know what you're doing clinically, but inside, you're questioning yourself. Am I doing this right?

Did I miss something?

Should I have done that differently?

That's normal, but no one really tells you that.

You're also not taught how to deal with the emotional side of the job. The things you see. The things you hear. The things that stay with you. Or how to handle difficult conversations. Or conflict. Or speaking up when something doesn't feel right. A lot of that you learn on the job. Through experience. Through mistakes. Through reflection. And through the people around you.

One thing that makes a huge difference is the team. A supportive team can build you up. Help you grow. Guide you. Give you confidence.

Over time, things start to click. You become more comfortable. More confident. More sure of yourself. But it doesn't happen overnight. You're never fully ready, and that's okay. Responsibility feels different when it's yours. Confidence builds with time and experience. It's normal to question yourself. The emotional side of nursing is real. A good team makes a huge difference. And learning doesn't stop after qualification.

Confidence, It Doesn't Come Overnight

People think you either have confidence or you don't. But in nursing, it doesn't work like that. Confidence is built slowly, over time.

When you first start, you might not feel confident at all. You double-check everything. You ask questions constantly. You replay situations in your head. And sometimes you compare yourself to others, more experienced nurses, people who seem like they have everything under control.

What you don't see is that they were once where you are. No one starts off confident. Confidence comes from doing. From repetition. From experience. From making decisions and learning from them. Even from making mistakes.

Every shift teaches you something. Every situation adds to your understanding. And slowly, without even realising it, you start to trust yourself. You walk onto the ward differently. You speak with more certainty. You make decisions with more clarity.

That doesn't mean you know everything; you never will. It means you know enough. And you know when to ask for help. Because confidence isn't about knowing it all. It's about knowing your limits. And being comfortable within them.

There will still be moments where you doubt yourself. That never fully goes away. But the difference is, you don't let it stop you. Confidence in nursing is closely linked to competence and safe practice. Confidence should never replace safe practice; it should support it.

The First Time You Lead a Shift

The first time you're in charge of a shift, you don't forget it. Even if no one makes a big deal about it. Even if it's just written next to your name on the rota. You feel it. Because suddenly, it's on you.

You're not just looking after your own patients anymore. You're looking at the whole ward. Staffing. Patient safety. Incidents. Decisions. Everything comes through you.

I remember that feeling. Walking onto the ward and knowing I'm the one in charge today. Even if there were more experienced staff around. Even if support was there. The responsibility still sat with me. And it's a different kind of pressure.

You start thinking differently. You're more aware. More alert. You become more conscious of everything happening around you. You're not just reacting anymore. You're anticipating. Who might need support? Where things could escalate. What needs to be prioritised? And at the same time, you're still doing your own job. It can feel like a lot.

There will be moments where you doubt yourself. Am I making the right decision? Should I have done that differently? That's normal. Because leadership isn't something you're suddenly perfect at. It's something you grow into.

You learn how to delegate. How to trust your team. How to ask for help when needed. And one of the biggest lessons? You don't have to do everything yourself. A good leader doesn't carry the whole shift alone. They use the team. They communicate. They listen.

Over time, you become more comfortable. That feeling of pressure doesn't disappear, but it becomes manageable. You start to trust your judgement. You start to find your rhythm. And one day, you realise you're not as nervous as you used to be.

Speaking Up, Finding Your Voice as a Nurse

Speaking up sounds simple. But it's not always easy, especially at the start of your career.

You're new. You're finding your feet. You don't want to say the wrong thing. You don't want to challenge someone more senior. So sometimes, you stay quiet. Even when something doesn't feel right.

I've been there. That moment when you notice something. Or you disagree with a decision. Or you feel something could be done differently. And there's that hesitation. Should I say something? Because speaking up can feel uncomfortable.

Over time, you realise something important. Your voice matters. Not because you know everything. But because you're part of the team. Because you see things. Because you're involved in patient care. And sometimes, you might be the one who notices something others haven't.

Speaking up isn't about challenging for the sake of it. It's about safety. Patient safety. Staff safety. Good practice.

Yes, it takes confidence. But it also takes courage. You don't have to be confrontational. You don't have to have all the answers. Sometimes it's as simple as saying, "Can I just check something?" Or, "I'm not sure about this." Or, "Can we look at this again?" Small things, but they matter. Because silence can be risky.

I've learned over the years that it's better to speak up and be wrong than stay quiet and regret it later.

As you grow in your role, it becomes easier. You find your voice. You trust your judgement. You become more comfortable having those conversations. And you encourage others to do the same. Because a good team is one where everyone feels able to speak.

Speaking up is a key part of safe and effective practice. Failure to speak up can compromise patient safety, allow poor practice to continue, and increase the risk of harm. A culture of openness supports safer care for everyone.

What Makes a Good Nurse?

What makes a good nurse? It's a question people ask a lot. After all these years, I don't think there's just one answer.

Being a good nurse isn't about one thing. Not just knowledge. Not just skills. Not just experience. It's a combination.

You can be clinically brilliant, know every medication, understand every condition, but if you can't connect with people, something is missing. And on the other hand, you can be the kindest person in the world. Caring. Compassionate. Supportive. But if you don't keep your knowledge up to date, that's a risk too.

So it's about balance.

For me, one of the most important things is care. Genuine care. Not just doing the job, but actually caring about the person in front of you. Patients can tell. They know when you're present. They know when you're just going through the motions.

Another thing is communication. How you speak. How you listen. How do you explain? Sometimes it's not what you say, it's how you say it. You can de-escalate a situation just by your tone. You can build trust just by listening.

Then there's accountability. Owning your actions. Doing things properly. Speaking up when something isn't right. No shortcuts. Because this job carries responsibility.

Teamwork is another big one. No one works alone in nursing. You rely on your team. You support each other. You communicate. A good nurse knows how to work with others, not against them.

Then there's resilience. Because this job will test you. Emotionally. Physically. Mentally. There will be hard days. Days that drain you. Days that stay with you. Being a good nurse doesn't mean those days don't affect you. It means you find a way to keep going, in a healthy way.

Boundaries matter too. Knowing where to draw the line. Being kind but professional. Supportive but not over-involved.

And finally, willingness to learn. No matter how long you've been in the job, you never know everything. Things change. Practice evolves. New challenges come. A good nurse keeps learning. Keeps growing.

Keeps reflecting. Because the moment you think you know it all, that's when things start to slip.

Looking back over my career, the nurses I've respected the most weren't perfect. But they were kind. Safe. Honest. Reliable. Willing to learn. And that, to me, is what makes a good nurse.

Am I a good nurse? I'll leave that one to my colleagues to answer.

Teamworking, What COVID Showed Me

I know I've spoken about teamworking already, but something came back to me. COVID.

When the pandemic hit, everything changed. No one really knew what to expect. There was uncertainty. Fear. Constant changes. What stood out to me the most was the team.

I've always believed in teamwork. I've worked in good teams throughout my career. But what I saw during COVID was something else. People came together in a way I hadn't seen before. Staff supporting each other. Stepping in without being asked. Covering shifts. Checking in on one another. There was this unspoken understanding that we're in this together. It didn't matter as much about roles. Everyone just did what needed to be done.

Working on COVID units wasn't easy. The PPE alone. Wearing full protective equipment for long periods. Masks. Visors. Gowns. It was uncomfortable. Draining. At times, overwhelming. But people kept going.

What amazed me the most was the attitude. Even in the middle of all that, people still showed care. Still showed compassion. Still showed up for patients, and for each other.

That's where you really see teamwork. Not when things are running smoothly, but when things are difficult. That's where you see the passion for nursing.

It made me realise something. We don't always give ourselves enough credit. We deal with a lot in this job. Every day. But during COVID, it was on another level. And still, people showed up. Nurses showed up. That's something I don't think should be forgotten.

When I look back on that time, what stands out to me isn't just how hard it was. It's how people came together. It was amazing to see.

Where It All Started

I wasn't sure at first whether to include this. I kept going back and forth in my head, do I put this in, or do I leave it out and just focus on the job, the nursing, the experiences on the ward?

But the truth is, this is part of me. This is where it all started.

I grew up in a country far from where I now work. Some of my earliest memories aren't very clear, but certain moments have stayed with me. Not because I understood them at the time, but because of how they felt.

I had a grandmother who wasn't well. As a young child, I didn't have the language for it. I didn't know what mental illness was. I didn't understand diagnoses, symptoms or behaviours. I just knew something wasn't right.

There were times I would see her, and something about her presence felt different. Not in a way I could explain. Just a feeling that stayed with me. Confusion, more than anything.

I remember my mum trying. Trying to get her help. Trying to find answers. She would take her to different places, speak to different people, searching for something, anything, that might make a difference.

But where I come from, mental illness wasn't always seen through a medical lens. People spoke about it in spiritual terms. In terms of forces and influences that today might sound unfamiliar. It wasn't unusual. It was part of the belief system, part of how people tried to make sense of things they couldn't explain. As a child, I didn't question it. I accepted what I heard, even if deep down it didn't quite sit right.

I just watched. And I wondered.

As I grew older, that curiosity never really left me. If anything, it grew stronger. I found myself wanting to understand what I had seen as a child. Wanting to put meaning to something that, for so long, didn't make sense. That curiosity is what led me into mental health nursing.

At the time, I don't think I fully realised just how much my past had influenced that decision. I thought I was just choosing a career. Looking back now, it feels like I was trying to find answers.

I remember being a student nurse, sitting in lectures, learning about different diagnoses. Schizophrenia. Psychosis. Catatonia. Listening to symptoms being described. Watching case studies. Reading through presentations. And then something clicked. It wasn't sudden, but it was clear.

I remember sitting there thinking, " This sounds familiar. Too familiar. And then it hit me. My grandmother.

For the first time, I started to piece things together. All those moments from childhood, all those things I didn't understand, they began to take shape. I can't say for certain what her diagnosis was. I'm not a doctor, and she was never formally assessed in a way I would recognise today. But from what I learned, paranoid schizophrenia, possibly with catatonic features, made sense to me. And that realisation stayed with me.

At one point, while I was still a student, I tried to reach out for advice. I spoke to a psychiatrist, hoping for some kind of guidance. Maybe clarity. Maybe reassurance that what I was thinking made sense. I didn't expect miracles. But I also didn't expect the response I got.

I remember being asked, "Have you tried going down the traditional route? The route of the old beliefs?"

It took me aback. I didn't know how to respond in that moment. Part of me was confused. Part of me was disappointed. And if I'm being honest, part of me felt heartbroken. Because deep down, I was hoping for something different. Something grounded in understanding. In care. In science. Not something that took me back to the same place my family had already been.

It made me realise something quite early on in my journey, that even within healthcare, there isn't always certainty. There isn't always a clear answer. And sometimes, even professionals can fall back on explanations that don't quite align with what you believe or hope for.

There wasn't much I could do at the time. I was still a student. Still learning. Still trying to find my place in all of this. And life, as it does, carried on.

My grandmother eventually passed away. But she never really left my story. Not in the way that matters.

Even now, as I reflect on my journey into mental health nursing, I can see her influence in ways I didn't recognise before. She was there at the beginning. In the confusion. In the questions. In the need to understand. In many ways, she shaped the nurse I was going to become.

When I look at patients now, when I see someone who is psychotic, withdrawn, distressed, or misunderstood, I don't just see symptoms. I see a person. I see someone's mother. Someone's grandmother. Someone's family. And without even realising it sometimes, a part of me goes back to her. Back to those early moments of not understanding, and wanting to.

Maybe that's what this job really is, for me. Not just caring. Not just managing risk or administering medication. But trying, in some small way, to give others the understanding that my grandmother never truly had.

When the Roles Change

Transitioning from staff nurse to management, that's a tricky one. And if I'm being honest, it's not something you can fully understand unless you've actually gone through it.

I've had a couple of those career transitions. The kind where you're working alongside someone, they might even be your manager at the time, and then suddenly, things change. You go for the role. You interview. You get the position. And just like that, the roles are reversed.

One of the most difficult situations is when someone has been acting up in that management role before you officially step into it. Because now, you're not just stepping into a new job. You're stepping into their space. You've worked together. You've built a certain dynamic. There's an unspoken understanding of who leads and who follows. And then overnight, that changes.

I remember one particular experience clearly. I walked into an office one day and found a conversation in progress, about me. It wasn't said directly to me, but I knew. You can tell.

I didn't challenge it at the time. I just took it in and carried on. In those moments, you realise very quickly what kind of situation you're stepping into.

Not long after, I had to do supervision. That's where it really becomes real. You're sitting across from someone you used to work alongside as equals, and now you're in a position where you're leading that conversation.

I remember saying something quite simple, but important. "Look, the roles are reversed now. But at the end of the day, I'm here to support you." And I meant that. For me, management was never about power. It was about responsibility.

It wasn't easy. There was resistance at first, and that's normal. People don't always adjust straight away. There can be tension, unspoken feelings, maybe even a bit of resentment. You feel it. Even when nothing is said directly, you feel it.

But over time, I've learned this: if you stay consistent, stay professional, and genuinely treat people with respect, things can change.

And they did. That same colleague, over time, began to accept the situation. The dynamic shifted again, this time in a healthier way. Eventually, we became good friends. Life happened, as it does. Different roles, different places, different paths, we lost touch. But that experience stayed with me. Because it taught me that difficult beginnings don't always mean difficult endings.

I've had similar situations happen more than once. Each time comes with its own challenges. But one thing I've always been conscious of is staying professional. I've never asked for people to be moved to different wards or units just to make things easier for me. It's tempting, sometimes. But I've always believed that part of leadership is learning how to work through challenges, not avoid them.

Management is an interesting one. When most of us become nurses, we don't do it to sit in offices or manage teams. We do it for the patients. That's what drew me in, anyway. But as you grow, personally and professionally, things change. You start thinking about progression. Sometimes it's financial. Sometimes it's about challenge. Sometimes it's other people encouraging you. "You'd be a good manager." "Why don't you go for it?" Eventually, you do.

I went for it. Ward manager. Then beyond that. Like anything, it comes with its positives and its challenges. I've enjoyed my management roles. They've taught me a lot, especially about people. That's the biggest lesson. You can think you know how to deal with people until you're in a position where you have to. Different personalities. Different expectations. Different pressures. Leadership isn't just about making decisions; it's about navigating people.

My toughest role was at the most senior level; different organisations give it different titles, but whatever you call it, it's a heavy role. That was probably the most challenging position I've held. You're not just managing a ward anymore. You're overseeing services, staff, systems, everything. The responsibility doesn't switch off. You're on call. Always. Even when you're not physically at work, you're mentally there.

There were times I had to be called in to deal with situations. Difficult situations. The kind you can't really prepare for, you just respond. I won't go into detail. Confidentiality matters. But that role tests you.

And still, I enjoyed it.

After some years, though, I realised something. I missed the patients. The higher up you go, the further away you get from the people you came into the profession for in the first place. Less contact. Less interaction. More meetings. More paperwork. Something in me felt that shift.

So I made a decision. I went back. Back onto the floor. Not because I couldn't do the role. But because I knew what mattered to me. I went back to working closely with patients again. Eventually stepping back into a ward manager role, but this time, with a different perspective.

Now, I make sure I stay involved. Daily. Present. Visible. Working alongside patients, not just overseeing from a distance. That's why I became a nurse.

Maybe that's what management really taught me. Not just how to lead people, but how not to lose yourself in the process.

When Silence Speaks Loudest

You don't expect it at first. You expect pressure. You expect stress. You expect the long shifts, the unpredictable patients, the emotional weight that follows you home. What you don't always expect is conflict within your own team.

And not the obvious kind. Not shouting. Not open arguments. The quiet kind. The kind where two staff members stop speaking to each other completely.

I've seen it happen more than once. Two colleagues, both good nurses, both competent, both dedicated, fall out. Sometimes it starts over something small. A disagreement in handover. A decision about a patient. A comment that was taken the wrong way. Sometimes it's deeper than that. But what follows is always the same. Silence.

At first, it's subtle. They stop making eye contact. Communication becomes short, direct, and only when absolutely necessary. They won't hand over properly to each other. Information is passed through someone else instead of being passed directly.

You notice it, but you think it'll pass. Sometimes it doesn't. That's when it starts affecting more than just them. Because in nursing, especially in mental health, communication isn't optional. It's safety.

I remember one shift where this exact situation was unfolding. Two members of staff had clearly fallen out. No one said it outright, but you could feel it in the atmosphere. The tension sat in the room. Heavy.

During handover, one of them spoke; the other didn't even look up. Information was missed. Small things at first, observations, changes in presentation, medication given earlier in the day. Things that might seem minor on the surface. In our environment, they matter. Everything matters.

As the shift went on, it became more obvious. They avoided working in the same space. If one were in the office, the other would stay on the floor. If one needed something, they'd ask someone else instead of going directly. It slows everything down.

And worse than that, it creates risk. Because when communication breaks down, gaps appear. And in those gaps, things get missed.

The hardest part is that both people are still doing their jobs. They're still caring for patients. Still completing tasks. Still showing up. But they're not working as a team anymore. And nursing is never an individual job.

As the nurse in charge, you feel it more. Because now you're not just managing the ward, you're managing the atmosphere. You start compensating without even realising it. Passing messages between them. Double-checking things that should have been handed over. Keeping an extra eye on everything because you don't fully trust that communication is flowing the way it should.

It's draining.

At some point, it has to be addressed. Avoiding it doesn't fix it. Time doesn't always fix it. I remember having to sit both staff members down separately first. Not to take sides. Not to assign blame. Just to understand. Because there are always two perspectives. Two experiences of the same situation. Usually, somewhere in the middle is the truth.

Then comes the harder part. Bringing it into the open. Encouraging a conversation that neither of them wants to have. It's uncomfortable. It's tense. Sometimes it feels like you're forcing something that shouldn't need to be forced. But it's necessary. Because at the end of the day, this isn't about friendship. It's about professionalism. It's about patient care.

I've said it before in those situations, and I'll say it again: "You don't have to like each other. But you do have to work together."

Most of the time, something shifts. Not always a full resolution. Not always an apology. But an agreement. A line drawn. A reset, even if it's just on the surface. Sometimes, that's enough.

I won't pretend it's easy. These situations linger. They affect morale. They affect trust. And if not handled properly, they can divide a team quietly over time.

In mental health nursing, we rely on each other just as much as we rely on our clinical skills. We walk into unpredictable situations. We manage risk constantly. We make decisions that can have serious consequences. We do that as a team. When that team fractures, even slightly, you feel it everywhere. In the handovers. In the ward atmosphere. In the way people support each other, or don't.

The patients notice too. They might not understand the details, but they feel the tension. They pick up on the disconnect. And in a setting where stability matters, that kind of energy can have an impact.

Working in a team isn't just about being skilled. It's about communication. Respect. Professional boundaries. And sometimes, putting personal feelings aside for the bigger picture. Because this job was never meant to be done alone. And silence, in the wrong places, can be louder than anything else.

Differences in People

I sat with this one for a long time. Longer than I expected to. I kept asking myself, " Does this belong in the book? Or is it something I leave out? Because once you say it, it's there. And once it's there, people will have opinions.

But this book was never meant to be filtered. It's about what I've seen. What I've felt. What I've learned along the way. And this is part of that journey.

Healthcare is one of the most diverse environments you can work in. You walk onto a ward, and you'll meet people from all over the world, different cultures, different accents, different upbringings, different ways of seeing things. Most of the time, that diversity is something special. You learn from each other. You adapt. You grow. You realise there isn't just one way to be a nurse.

Alongside that, though, there are things that don't always get spoken about. Things that sit quietly in the background.

A lot of migrants work in healthcare. That's the reality. People leave their home countries, their families, everything familiar, and come into a system that is already demanding, already stretched, already emotionally heavy. On top of that, sometimes, they face things that others don't.

Racism is one of those things. And it doesn't always come in the way people expect. It's not always someone saying something outright. It's not always something you can easily report or prove. Sometimes it's in the way people are treated differently. Sometimes it's in who gets listened to and who doesn't. Sometimes it's in who gets opportunities and who gets overlooked.

I've seen situations where someone was clearly ready to step into a higher role. A person of colour, experienced, capable, and respected by the team. Someone who knew the job inside out. Someone who could lead. When the opportunity came, they didn't get it. Someone else did.

I'm not saying every situation like that is racism. That wouldn't be fair. But when you see it happen more than once and start noticing patterns, you can't help but question it. Even if you never say it out loud.

I remember someone asking me about it once. "Why didn't you say something?" I understood the question. From the outside, it can look simple: just speak up. But in reality, it's not always that straightforward. Not every situation is clear-cut. Not every moment is yours to step into. Not every environment feels safe enough to challenge something like that openly.

I'm not someone who stays quiet when something is clearly wrong. If I need to speak, I will. But I've also learned that timing matters. Position matters. And sometimes, the impact of speaking isn't always what you think it will be. That doesn't mean it's right. It just means it's complicated.

The truth is, these things happen. Not just in nursing. Not just in healthcare. But because healthcare has such a high number of migrant workers, you notice it more. You hear different stories. You see different experiences. Some people talk about it openly. Others don't. Some don't even realise it's happening to them. That's the part that really makes you stop and think.

As for me, have I experienced racism? Yes, and no. Nothing has completely shaken me. Nothing has defined my career. But small things. Moments. Comments. Situations where you pause for a second and think, was that because of…? And then you move on. Because you have a job to do. Patients to look after. Responsibilities to carry. A role that doesn't stop for reflection in the middle of a shift.

I've always been grounded in who I am. I know the kind of person I am. I know how I treat people. So I've never allowed my skin colour to define my worth. If someone else chooses to judge based on that, that's something they need to answer for, not me.

That doesn't mean it should be ignored. This book isn't about calling things out or challenging systems directly. It's not about making statements or leading debates. It's about sharing experiences. The real ones. The uncomfortable ones as well as the good. This is one of those uncomfortable truths. Something that exists in the background of many workplaces. Not always visible. Not always acknowledged. But there.

What I've noticed over the years is that people deal with it in very different ways. Some people challenge it head-on. Some people report it. Some people speak openly about their experiences. Some people carry it quietly. There's no single right way. Everyone has their own threshold. Their own circumstances. Their own way of protecting themselves.

What I do know is this: it takes strength to walk into a system that isn't always built with you in mind, and still show up every day. To still care. To still give. To still do your job to a high standard.

I've worked with so many people like that. Strong, capable, dedicated individuals who bring so much to the profession. People who deserve recognition. People who deserve opportunities. People who deserve to be seen for what they truly bring, not judged on anything else.

The Shift That Never Ended

I remember one shift I worked, years ago, in a hospital where we ran early, late, and night shifts. It was winter, and not just any winter; it was brutal. The kind where everything feels harder before the day even begins.

That morning, my day started off wrong. My car wouldn't start.

Straight away, stress. I rang the ward to let them know I'd be a bit late. Tried calling a colleague to see if they could pick me up, but no luck. So I had no choice but to get the bus.

By the time I arrived at work, I already felt flustered. Nothing could have prepared me for what I was about to walk into.

As soon as I opened the door onto the unit, a book came flying towards me. I had to duck. To this day, I don't think it was meant for me. I just happened to be walking in at the wrong moment. But that's how it is sometimes. You step into it without warning.

I moved quickly towards the office near the entrance, heart racing.

The unit was in chaos. Patients shouting. Staff are trying to de-escalate. Alarms are going off. People talking over each other. That kind of noise that isn't just loud. It's overwhelming.

It was mayhem.

I dropped my bag and went straight back out. No time to think. No time to settle in. Straight into restraint. And not just one. There were two, maybe three patients in restraints at the same time. Staff stretched, trying to manage everything safely. You don't think in those moments. You react. You rely on your training, your team, and your instincts.

Time disappears. I couldn't tell you how long it lasted. Minutes feel like seconds and seconds feel like minutes. Everything happens so fast. At one point, I had to be relieved by another staff member, because you physically can't keep going forever.

Eventually, things began to settle. Then came the part no one really prepares you for, the paperwork. The incident report. Where do you even begin?

Back then, it was all paper-based. No computers. Just a form and a pen. I ended up writing one report for all three restraints. Later on, management came back to me and said I could have written separate ones. But honestly, none of us could even remember the exact details. During the debrief, we couldn't recall who held which arm, who was on which leg. All we knew was this. There were three patients in restraints. We kept people safe. We got through it.

That shift didn't really slow down after that. An early shift runs from around half seven to half two or three, but that day felt like a full twenty-four hours packed into a few. It was relentless.

What stayed with me most didn't happen during the chaos. It happened after.

The debrief was quick. Too quick, if I'm honest. I remember thinking, we just went through all of that together.

So I did something small. I got bits of paper and wrote little notes to each staff member involved. Just simple things. Thank you. Well done. I appreciate you.

I folded them and handed them out to people as they left the shift. To me, it was nothing big. Just being me. Just acknowledging the team. But the response was that people genuinely appreciated it.

Then, years later, about five years ago, something happened that I'll never forget.

One of the staff from that shift somehow got my number. They sent me a message. Attached was a photo of that note. They told me they had kept it all those years. They said they had never felt so appreciated before.

I cried. Because to me, it was such a small thing. But to them, it meant everything.

That moment taught me something I carry to this day: never underestimate the power of appreciation.

Even now, I still do it. I'll send a quick message after a shift. Thanks for today. Great job. Really appreciated your support. Because it matters more than we realise.

***

After that shift, I went home, had a shower, and went straight to bed. I was shattered.

At some point, I woke up. It was dark. Now, it was winter, so darkness didn't mean much. I didn't check the time. I just assumed I had slept through the night.

Panic kicked in. I got dressed quickly, called a taxi, and rushed back to work.

When I arrived, I walked into the office. Everyone looked at me, strangely.

I sat down and said, "Guys, I'm so sorry I'm late." They just stared at me. Someone said, "What do you mean?" I said, "I'm late."

That's when they said it. "You're not supposed to be here. You were on an early shift. You were here this morning."

I had gone home so exhausted, slept for just a few hours, and convinced myself it was the next day. I had come back in for the late shift on the same day.

We all laughed. What else could you do?

I went back home, got into bed again, and came back properly the next day.

That shift taught me a lot. About pressure. About teamwork. About gratitude. And about just how exhausted this job can make you.

More than anything, it reminded me that the work doesn't always end when the shift does. Sometimes it follows you home. Sometimes it wakes you up in the dark and sends you out the door. And sometimes, only sometimes, it gives something back, in a folded piece of paper somebody has kept for five years.

That's the job. That's all of it, really.

Part One, The Weight You Don't Expect

Chapter 1
After the Shift

Sitting in the car again.

Engine off.

Just silence.

It's strange how the day doesn't really end when the shift finishes. Hand over, you clock out, walk out the doors… but your mind is still inside.

Still on the ward.

I keep replaying little moments.

Things I said.

Things I didn't say.

That patient who didn't seem right, even though everything looked "fine" on paper.

You tell yourself you've done your job. That you handed everything over properly. That the next team will pick it up.

But still… it lingers.

I think that's the part people don't see.

They think once you leave, that's it. You go home, switch off, and carry on like anyone else after work.

But it doesn't quite work like that.

You carry pieces with you.

A conversation.

A look someone gave you.

A feeling you can't quite shake.

Sometimes it's heavy. Sometimes it's just there in the background.

Today… I don't even know what it is.

Just tired, I think.

Not just physically. That kind of tired you can't really sleep off.

I sat here longer than I needed to.

Didn't rush to go anywhere.

Just needed a moment where no one needed anything from me.

No questions.

No decisions.

No responsibility.

Just quiet.

I suppose that's how I reset.

Before going home.

Before stepping back into normal life.

Or at least… what's meant to feel like normal.

Chapter 2
The Things You Carry Home

There's something about this job that people don't always understand.

You don't just leave it at work.

You carry it home.

Not physically.

But mentally.

Emotionally.

Sometimes even quietly, without realising it.

You finish your shift, you walk out of the ward, you get into your car or on the bus, and on the outside… it looks like you've switched off.

But inside?

You're still there.

Still thinking.

Still replaying.

Still holding things

I've lost count of how many times I've gone home and sat in silence, just going over the day.

Thinking about patients

Conversations.

Things that were said.

Things that weren't said.

Wondering if I handled something the right way.

Wondering if I could have done more.

That's the part that stays with you.

Not always the big incidents.

Sometimes it's the small things.

A look someone gave you.

A patient opening up.

Someone crying.

Someone is not talking at all.

Those moments don't just disappear.

They sit with you.

And you carry them.

I remember times when I'd be at home, with my family, and my mind would drift back to work.

Not because I wanted it to.

But because it just does.

You think about whether someone is okay.

Whether they settled after you left.

Whether the night staff had a better shift.

Whether something escalated.

You don't always get closure in this job.

You hand over, and you go.

But the thoughts don't always go with you.

And that can be heavy.

Especially in mental health.

Because you're not just dealing with tasks.

You're dealing with people's lives.

Their trauma.

Their struggles.

Their pain.

And when someone shares that with you, you don't just forget it.

You hold it.

Even if you don't realise you are.

I think when I first started, I didn't fully understand that.

I thought once I left work, that was it.

But over time, I realised, it doesn't work like that.

You learn to manage it.

You have to.

Because if you don't, it builds up.

And it can affect you.

Your mood.

Your energy.

Even though you show up at home.

There were times I'd come home and be quieter than usual.

Not because anything was wrong at home.

But because I was still processing the day.

Still carrying things I hadn't put down yet.

And sometimes, you don't even have the words to explain it.

Because how do you explain what you've seen?

What have you heard?

How do you switch from that… to normal life?

It's not always easy.

And I think that's something people don't always talk about.

The emotional weight of the job.

Not just during the shift, but after it.

The invisible part.

The part no one sees.

You might look fine.

You might say, "Yeah, work was okay."

But inside, you're still holding a lot.

Over time, I learned that you have to find ways to let it go.

Or at least… not let it sit so heavily.

For some people, it's talking.

For others, it's writing.

For some, it's just having quiet time to decompress.

There's no one way.

But there has to be something.

Because carrying everything, all the time, isn't sustainable.

And yet, we do it.

Without even thinking.

Because we care.

Because we connect.

Because we're human.

And that's the balance in this job.

Caring enough to do it well.

But not carrying so much that it breaks you.

I'm still learning that balance.

I think most of us are.

Some days you manage it well.

Other days, it follows you home a bit more than you'd like.

And that's okay.

Because this job isn't just a job.

It's something you feel.

Something you experience.

Something that becomes part of you.

But it's important to remember —

It doesn't have to become all of you.

You're allowed to put it down.

You're allowed to switch off.

You're allowed to have a life outside of it.

Even if sometimes…

It takes a bit longer to get there.

Chapter 3
The Things You Never Say Out Loud

There are things you learn in this job that never make it into training.

Not because they're not important.

But because they're not the kind of things people want to admit.

Even to themselves.

Especially not out loud.

You learn very quickly what you're supposed to say.

How to speak to patients. How to document. How to present things in a way that sounds professional, measured, and appropriate.

And you do that.

You get good at it.

But underneath all of that—there's another layer.

The thoughts that don't make it into notes.

The feelings that don't get discussed in handover.

The moments where you catch yourself thinking something and immediately push it down because… you're not supposed to think like that.

But you do.

We all do.

You just don't say it.

There are days when you feel nothing.

And that's probably one of the hardest things to admit.

You're standing there, talking to someone who is clearly struggling, clearly in pain, and you're doing everything right on the outside—listening, responding, supporting.

But inside… It's quiet.

Too quiet.

And you start questioning yourself.

What's wrong with me?

Because you remember a time when you would have felt it. When it would have stayed with you long after your shift ended.

Now, sometimes, it doesn't.

And instead of relief, there's a kind of guilt that comes with that.

Like you've lost something you weren't supposed to lose.

But at the same time, you know—if you felt everything, all the time, you wouldn't last.

So you learn to balance it.

Or at least, you try.

There are moments when you look at the system and quietly think:

This isn't working.

You don't say it in meetings.

You don't write it in reports.

But you feel it.

When the same patients come back again and again.

When decisions are made that make sense on paper, but don't sit right in reality.

When you know there's more someone needs—but it's just not there to give.

And you carry that.

Because you're part of it.

Even when you don't fully agree with it.

There are times you feel frustrated.

Not at the patients—but at the situation.

At the cycle.

The feeling that no matter how much effort goes in, the outcome doesn't always change.

And that frustration… You keep it to yourself.

Because it's not something people like to hear.

It doesn't fit the image of what this job is supposed to be.

There are days when you're tired in a way that has nothing to do with sleep.

Where it's not your body that's worn out—it's something deeper.

And someone asks, "Are you okay?"

And you say, "Yeah, I'm fine."

Because explaining it would take too long.

And even then, you're not sure you could put it into words properly.

There are moments when you second-guess yourself.

A decision you made. Something you said. Something you didn't say.

You go over it again and again, wondering if there was a better way to handle it.

If you missed something.

If you could have made a difference.

And you don't always get an answer.

Sometimes it just sits with you.

Unresolved.

There are things you see that don't leave you.

Not in an obvious way.

Not like a dramatic memory you can clearly point to.

But in small flashes.

A face. A moment. A sentence someone said.

And it comes back to you at random times, when you're not expecting it.

Sitting at home. Driving. Trying to switch off.

And for a second, you're right back there.

And then it passes.

But it never fully goes.

There are also moments—quiet ones—where you question how long you can keep doing it.

Not in a dramatic, "I'm leaving" kind of way.

Just a thought that crosses your mind.

Can I keep carrying this?

And then the next day comes, and you go back.

Because that's what you do.

You show up.

Even with all of that sitting in the background.

And maybe the biggest thing you never say out loud is this:

You don't have all the answers.

You're not always sure you're making the right call.

You don't always feel as steady as you appear.

But you keep going anyway.

You learn to hold all of it at once.

The compassion and the detachment

The frustration and the understanding.

The doubt and the responsibility.

And you carry it quietly.

Because that's the part of the job people don't really see.

Not the obvious moments.

Not the crises.

But the internal weight of it.

The thoughts you manage.

The feelings you regulate.

The things you never say—

But live with it every day.

And maybe that's what shapes you the most.

Not what happens in front of you.
But everything that stays inside.

Chapter 4
Do Nurses Have Favourite Patients?

It's a question people don't usually ask out loud.

But you can see it in their eyes sometimes.

In the way they watch you interact.

In the way they measure your tone, your patience, your softness.

Do nurses have favourites?

Are the favourites the ones who say 'please' and 'thank you'?

The ones who don't ring the bell every ten minutes?

The ones who apologise for being sick, as if illness is an inconvenience to us?

Or is it the opposite?

Is it the difficult ones?

The loud ones, the ones who challenge you, who make you think, who make you feel something other than routine?

The ones who don't let you switch off?

Do nurses prefer the quiet patients?

The ones who fade into the background.

Who doesn't ask for much?

Who do you have to remind yourself to check on because they won't ask?

Or do those patients worry us more?

Do we lie awake thinking about the ones who say they're "fine" a little too quickly?

The ones who smile when nothing about their situation is okay?

Do we get attached?

To the man who tells the same story every morning like it's the first time.

To the woman who grips your hand just a little tighter when you say goodbye.

Is that favouritism?

Or is that just being human?

Do we treat them differently?

Do we spend more time in some rooms than in others?

Do we notice some absences more than others?

And if we do… does that make us better nurses, or worse ones?

Are favourites the ones who remind us of someone?

A father.

A sister.

A younger version of ourselves.

Is it easier to care when you can see a piece of your own life reflected back at you?

Or is it harder?

Do we protect ourselves from that?

Build quiet walls so that every patient gets the same version of us?

Measured. Professional. Fair.

Is fairness the same as equality?

Can care ever truly be equal when people are so different?

When some patients need more words, and others need silence.

When some need boundaries, and others need warmth.

Do nurses have favourites…

Or do certain patients just stay with us longer than others?

Long after the shift ends.

Long after the bed is filled by someone new.

Long after their name disappears from the board.

And if they stay…

What does that mean?

I ask these questions sometimes…

And I have asked myself: do I have, or have I ever had, favourite patients?

Part Two, The Realities of the Ward

Chapter 5
System Pressure

We don't always talk about it directly.

We mention it in passing, "we're short today", "it's busy". Little phrases that don't really capture what's actually going on.

But the pressure is always there.

Constant.

It's in the background of every shift.

You feel it before you even start. You walk onto the ward, and you already know what kind of day it's going to be. Not because anything has happened yet… but because of what's not there.

Not enough staff.

Not enough time.

You try not to let it affect how you work.

You still greet people properly. Still try to give time. Still try to listen. But there's always that quiet awareness in the back of your mind, you can't stay too long. There's something else waiting. Someone else needs something.

You move from one thing to the next.

Medication.

Observations.

Incidents.

Documentation.

And somewhere in between all that… you're supposed to care.

Proper care.

Not just tasks. Not just ticking boxes.

Actual care.

That's the hardest part.

Because the system sometimes pushes you towards doing the job… rather than being the nurse.

I've had days where I've walked away from a patient mid-conversation because something else urgent came up. And I remember thinking, that's not how this should be.

But what do you do?

There's no extra time hidden somewhere.

No extra staff suddenly appearing.

You just adjust. Prioritise. Re-prioritise. Keep going.

And then there are the beds, this is more in acute settings.

Always the beds.

Patients needing admission. No space. Pressure to discharge. Pressure to move people on.

Sometimes you find yourself asking, are we making this decision because it's the right time for the patient… or because we need the bed?

That's not a comfortable place to be.

But it's real.

And it's not about blaming anyone.

It's the system.

Managers are under pressure. Nurses are under pressure. Doctors are under pressure. Everyone is trying to make something work with what they have.

But sometimes what we have… isn't enough.

And that's where it becomes difficult.

Because you carry that with you.

The feeling that you could have done more if you had more time.

That someone needed a bit longer.

That something was missed, not because you didn't care, but because you couldn't stretch any further.

That's the kind of pressure that doesn't show on paper.

It doesn't get documented.

But it sits with you.

Shift after shift.

And still… You come back.

You put the uniform on again.

You walk back into the same environment.

You try again.

Because despite all of it, the pressure, the lack, the constant push, you still want to do right by people.

Even if the system doesn't always make it easy.

Chapter 6
Just the Two of Us

I remember one shift clearly.

We were meant to be five staff.

That was the number. That was what was considered safe. Manageable.

But that's not how the day went.

Three staff members rang in sick.

Just like that.

The agency couldn't provide anyone. Bank staff, the extra staff a ward can call on at short notice, couldn't come in. Regular staff didn't pick up overtime.

And suddenly… it was just two of us.

On a unit that was already difficult to manage on a good day.

Busy most of the time.

Incidents are not everyday, but they are often enough to keep you alert. Always watching. Always anticipating.

And that day… two staff.

I remember standing there at the start of the shift, thinking, how is this going to work?

Because what do you do in that situation?

We have a duty of care. You can't just put your tools down and say, "There's not enough of us, we're going home."

It doesn't work like that.

The patients are still there.

They still need care.

They still need support.

So, you stay.

You adjust.

You do what you can.

And you hope nothing goes wrong.

What people don't realise is... patients always know.

They watch us.

They see everything.

They notice when staffing is low, when things are stretched, when something isn't quite right.

They know.

And that day, they knew.

There's no word of a lie, something shifted.

It's hard to explain.

The two of us managed the whole unit.

No incidents.

Not one.

On a unit where incidents weren't unusual.

I remember looking around at different moments and noticing small things.

Patients regulating themselves.

You could see it, people breathing in and out, trying to manage their own distress. The kind of thing we normally have to step in and support with.

I remember asking one patient,

"Are you alright? Do you want to talk?"

And they said,

"No, it's okay. You go and do what you need to do."

Another one noticed the dinner trolley sitting there.

"I've seen the trolley, go and serve the food."

They helped.

Not in a formal way. Not because they were asked.

But because they understood.

Because they could see we were stretched.

And somehow… we got through the shift.

Just the two of us.

No incidents.

Everyone safe.

Everything done.

It doesn't make sense when you think about it.

Because by all standards, that situation wasn't safe. It shouldn't have worked.

But it did.

And it stayed with me.

Because in that moment, it reminded me of something we don't always say out loud, patients are more aware, more capable, and more human than they're often given credit for.

They saw us.

And in their own way… they supported us.

That doesn't take away from the reality of system pressures. It doesn't make it okay that we were left in that situation.

But it showed something else.

That even in the middle of pressure, risk, and not enough staff…

There can still be understanding.

There can still be a connection.

And sometimes, in the most unexpected moments…

People meet you halfway.

Chapter 7
The Revolving Door

There are some patients you expect to see again before they've even left.

Not because you want to.

But because, deep down, you know.

You go through the process the same as always—reviews, plans, conversations about progress, and discussions around discharge. Everything is done properly. Everything is documented. On paper, it makes sense.

They're stable enough. Safe enough. Ready enough.

And still, there's a part of you that isn't convinced.

You don't always say it out loud.

Sometimes there's no solid reason you can point to. No clear risk, no obvious concern that would justify keeping them in.

Just a feeling.

A quiet thought at the back of your mind:

We'll see them again.

And more often than not, you're right.

They leave.

And for a while, there's a kind of calm. The bed is free. The ward moves on. New admissions come in, new situations take over, and the pace doesn't slow down long enough for you to sit with it.

Until their name shows up again.

On the board. On the list. On the handover.

And there's a moment—small, but noticeable—where something sinks.

Not shock.

Not even frustration, exactly.

Just a kind of tired recognition.

They're back.

You see them come through the doors again, and sometimes they look exactly the same as when they left. Other times, they look worse. More worn down. More distant. Like something has taken a bit more out of them since the last time.

And you pick up where you left off.

Same conversations.

Same patterns.

Same attempts to move things forward.

You remind yourself that every admission is a chance. That progress isn't linear. That recovery takes time.

And all of that is true.

But there's another side to it.

The part that doesn't get said as often.

Because it does something to you, seeing the same cycle over and over again.

Admitted.

Stabilised.

Discharged.

Readmitted.

At some point, it starts to blur.

You struggle to separate one admission from the next. Conversations feel familiar before they've even happened. You find yourself finishing sentences in your head because you've heard them before.

And that's when the doubt creeps in.

Not about them.

About the process.

You start questioning whether what you're doing is actually helping—or just maintaining something that keeps repeating itself.

You wonder what happens in between admissions. What support is really there? What breaks down? What gets missed?

Because something is.

It has to be.

People don't keep coming back like that for no reason.

There was one patient in particular.

They came in so often that their presence felt almost routine. You'd hear their name and already know the general outline of what the admission would look like.

How they'd present.

What they'd say.

How would it progress?

And that familiarity—it's dangerous in a way.

Because you have to fight against it.

You have to remind yourself that even if you've seen it before, this is still their experience right now.

Not a repeat.

Not something to be rushed through because you think you know how it ends.

But it's hard.

Because part of you does know how it often ends.

Another discharge.

Another attempt.

Another return.

And each time, you notice small changes.

Not always improvements.

Sometimes, just wear.

On them.

And on you.

You become more cautious about optimism. More measured in what you expect. You stop looking for big changes and start focusing on smaller, quieter signs that something—anything—is different this time.

Sometimes it is.

Sometimes it isn't.

And that uncertainty stays with you.

Because you want it to work.

You want this admission to be the one that sticks. The one that breaks the cycle.

But you also learn not to hold onto that too tightly.

Because when it doesn't happen, when they come back again, there's a weight to that.

Not failure.

But something close enough to it that you feel it.

You don't talk about it much.

You just carry on.

Do the work.

Have the conversations again.

Offer the same support, even when it feels like you're retracing steps.

Because that's the job.

And maybe that's the reality of it.

That not every story moves forward in a straight line.

Some go in circles.

Some take longer.

Some come back again and again before anything truly changes—if it ever does.

And maybe the role isn't always to stop the cycle completely.

Maybe sometimes it's just to be there within it.

Consistently.

Without judgment.

Even when it's frustrating.

Even when it's tiring.

Even when part of you is quietly wondering if anything is really changing at all.

Because for them, each time isn't just a repeat.

It's another point where something wasn't manageable anymore.

Another moment where they needed somewhere to come back to.

And for better or worse, we were the place they came back to.

Chapter 8
The Ones With No One

There's always one that stays with you.

Not because they were the most unwell. Not because their story was the worst.

But because of what was left around them.

Or more accurately, what wasn't.

In mental health, you come across it more than people realise. Patients with no one. No family visiting. No friends calling. At some point, people drift away. Sometimes they can't cope. Sometimes they don't understand. Sometimes they've just had enough.

And you can't always blame them.

Mental illness doesn't just affect the person—it takes something from everyone around them too. It wears people down. It stretches patience. It changes relationships in ways that aren't always repairable.

I looked after one patient for a few years.

At the beginning, he had a family. They came in regularly, sat with him, and tried to support him. You could see they cared. You could see they were trying to hold on to who he was before all of this.

But then he relapsed.

Badly.

And something shifted.

The visits became less frequent. Shorter. More strained. Conversations that used to flow started to feel forced. You could see it happening, even if no one said it out loud.

Then eventually, they stopped coming altogether.

Before they disappeared completely, they made it clear—to him and to us—that they couldn't do it anymore. That's when he became unwell like this; they couldn't handle it. This admission… this was the last one for them.

I remember how final it sounded.

Not said in anger. Not even said coldly.

Just… done.

And then one day, they were gone.

No more visitors. No more familiar faces walking onto the ward. No one was asking how he was doing. No one was sitting beside him in silence just so he wasn't alone.

Just us.

You try to fill that space as a nurse, in whatever way you can. You spend a bit more time. You check in more often. You sit, even when there are a hundred other things to be doing.

But it's not the same.

It will never be the same.

There were times he would slip into deep depression. Heavy. The kind where he barely spoke, barely moved, barely engaged with anything around him.

And you knew.

It wasn't just the illness.

It was the absence of anyone waiting for him outside those walls.

That kind of loneliness is hard to explain.

It's not just being alone—it's knowing that no one is coming.

You could feel it around him sometimes. Almost like it had weight. Like it sat in the room with us. You'd walk in and sense it before a word was even said.

And no matter what we did, we couldn't take that part away.

That stays with you.

More than people would expect.

Because this job doesn't just end when your shift finishes.

It follows you home.

Not in obvious ways. Not in dramatic flashes.

It's quieter than that.

You sit down in the evening, trying to switch off, and your mind drifts back to the ward. To faces. To moments. To people like him.

You replay conversations. Wonder if you said the right thing. If you missed something. If there was more you could have done, even when you know, realistically, there wasn't.

You tell yourself to leave it at work.

That's what you're supposed to do.

But some things don't stay there.

They linger.

There was a time I could switch off. Or at least I think there was. Early on, I'd go home tired, maybe emotionally drained, but it didn't sit with me like this.

(removed sentence that was here)

Some days it's just a passing thought. Other days it's heavier. Harder to ignore.

You start noticing changes in yourself.

Small ones at first.

You become a bit more distant. A bit more guarded. You don't react the way you used to. Things that once would have stayed with you for days now barely register.

And at some point, you realise that's not because they matter less.

It's because you've learned how to shut parts of yourself off.

Or at least, you think you have.

Until something breaks through.

A moment. A patient. A memory.

And suddenly, everything you thought you'd packed away is right there again.

Clear as ever.

I still think about him.

More than I probably should.

I wonder where he is now. If he ever made it out of the hospital. If he managed to build something for himself. If anyone ever came back.

Or if he's still carrying that same silence with him.

Because moments like that stay with you—not because of what you did or didn't do.

But because you realise something you don't learn in training

There are parts of this job you can't fix

No matter how much time you give. No matter how much you care.

And maybe the hardest part is learning to sit with that.

Knowing that sometimes, all you can offer someone…

is that they're not completely alone in that moment.

Even if, outside those walls, no one is waiting.

Chapter 9
When the Allegation Comes

False accusations.

It's not something you think about when you first come into nursing. Or maybe you do, briefly, in training, mentioned in passing, tucked into policies and procedures.

But you don't really understand it until you see it happen.

I remember a few years after I qualified, a patient made an allegation against a member of staff.

I won't go into detail about what was said. That part almost becomes secondary over time. What stayed with me wasn't the allegation itself, it was what came after.

The impact.

Because once an allegation is made, everything changes.

It has to be taken seriously. That's the first thing. And rightly so. Patients must be protected. Their voices have to be heard, even when things are unclear.

So an investigation was started.

And just like that, the staff member was no longer just a colleague going about their shift, they became someone under scrutiny.

I remember thinking how quickly it all shifted.

One day, you're part of the team.

The next, you're at home… waiting.

The investigation took six weeks.

Six weeks doesn't sound long on paper. But when you're the one sitting at home, thinking about your career, your reputation, your future, six weeks stretches into something much heavier.

You can only imagine what goes through someone's mind during that time.

Replaying every interaction.

Questioning yourself.

Wondering how something like this even happened.

At the same time, on the ward, the patient was fully supported.

As they should be.

That's the balance that's hard to sit with, knowing both things have to happen at once. The patient must be protected and believed enough to investigate properly. And the staff member… well, they're left in a kind of limbo.

Not guilty. Not cleared. Just… suspended in uncertainty.

It's not an easy place to be.

I remember how it affected the team as well.

People became quieter. More cautious. More aware of how easily things can shift.

There's a kind of unspoken tension that creeps in when something like that is happening. You don't always talk about it openly, but it's there.

In the end, after six weeks, the allegation was found to be false.

The patient later retracted what they had said.

But by then, six weeks had already passed.

And even when something is resolved, it doesn't just disappear.

Something lingers.

That experience stayed with me because it highlighted how complex this work really is.

Sometimes patients make allegations because they are unwell. Their perception of reality is altered. What feels real to them may not have happened in the way it's described.

Other times, allegations are true.

And that's why every single one has to be taken seriously.

There's no easy way around it.

No shortcuts.

But that doesn't make it any easier for the people involved.

I've seen how these situations affect both sides.

The patient needs to be heard, protected, and supported.

The staff member is dealing with fear, uncertainty, and the weight of something that can change everything.

And the team, somewhere in the middle, is trying to hold both.

That's the part people don't always see.

The balancing.

The constant awareness of safety, for the patient, for your colleague, for yourself.

It makes you more careful.

More aware of boundaries.

More conscious of how you communicate, how you position yourself, and how you document. Not in a fearful way, but in a way that reminds you just how vulnerable everyone is in this environment.

I've been fortunate.

Touch wood, I've never had an allegation made against me.

But I've seen enough to know that it's always a possibility.

And that awareness never fully leaves you.

What I've learned from it all is this:

You have to support your patient.

You have to support your colleague.

And you have to make sure everyone is safe.

There's no picking sides.

Just doing your best to hold the situation with fairness, professionalism, and humanity.

It's not easy. It's tough.

But it's part of the reality of the job.

And like many things in nursing…

You only really understand it once you've seen it up close.

…………

Chapter 10
The Debate About Male and Female Wards

Male and female wards.

It sounds simple when you say it out loud. Like something already decided. Categorised. Neat.

But I remember a time when it didn't feel simple at all.

It must be over ten years ago now. Maybe more. One of those conversations that started casually, probably in the staff room, cups of tea going cold, someone leaning back in their chair throwing out a question that didn't seem like much at the time.

Should male staff only work on male psychiatric wards?

Should female staff only work on female wards?

At first, it felt like just another topic to pass the time. Something theoretical. But it didn't stay like that for long.

Everyone had something to say.

You could feel it shift, that moment when a conversation stops being light and starts meaning something. People sat up a bit straighter. Voices got firmer. The kind of discussion where you realise people aren't just talking… they're defending something.

My opinion was always the same.

If we're trying to normalise life for our patients, then why would we divide it so rigidly? The outside world doesn't work like that. Life isn't separated into male-only and female-only spaces in that way. People interact with everyone, different genders, different personalities, different dynamics.

So why would we create an environment that doesn't reflect that?

To me, having both male and female staff on a ward felt more real. More balanced. More like life outside those walls.

But that didn't sit right with everyone.

Some of my colleagues spoke about safety, and not in a vague way, but with weight behind it. Real concerns. Situations they had seen, or experienced. You couldn't dismiss that.

Others talked about boundaries. About vulnerability. About how certain patients might respond differently depending on who was caring for them.

And then there were those who didn't speak much at first, but when they did, you could tell it had been sitting with them for a long time.

The room changed.

What started as a discussion became something sharper. More personal.

I remember one colleague in particular. Quiet up until that point. Listening. Watching. And then suddenly they stood up.

Properly stood up.

And before anyone really had time to react, they slammed their hand down on the table.

The sound cut through everything.

It wasn't dramatic for the sake of it. It came from somewhere deeper. Frustration, maybe. Or conviction. Or something they'd been holding onto for a long time.

For a moment, nobody spoke.

You could feel it, that pause where everyone becomes aware that this isn't just a conversation anymore.

It mattered.

Funny thing is, I don't actually remember how it ended.

No big conclusion. No agreement. No resolution neatly tied up.

We just… went back to work.

Observations to finish. Medications to give. Patients to check on. As if the intensity of that moment could just be folded away and left behind in the staff room.

But it never really left.

I still think about it sometimes.

Not in a way that keeps me up at night, but in that quiet, passing way. Like something unfinished.

I still don't know if there's a right answer.

Maybe there isn't one.

Maybe it depends on the ward. The patients. The staff. The history that walks into the room with each person.

Or maybe the question was never really about male and female wards at all.

Maybe it was about how we try, and sometimes struggle, to balance safety with normality.

Protection with dignity.

Care with reality.

All I know is, for something that sounded so straightforward...

It never really was.

Chapter 11
It Happens Everywhere

No one tells you when you start nursing that you're not just walking into a job.

You're walking into a whole little world of its own.

A place where people spend more time with each other than they do with their own families. Long shifts, weekends, holidays—you end up seeing the same faces over and over again, in every possible mood. Tired, stressed, laughing, barely holding it together.

And over time, something happens.

People connect.

Sometimes in the normal ways—friendships, support, having someone to get you through a rough shift.

And sometimes… in other ways.

It's part of life, I suppose.

But no one really prepares you for how common it is.

Or how obvious it becomes.

You don't notice it straight away when you're new. You're too busy trying to survive your shift, figure out what you're doing, and not make a mistake.

But give it time.

You start to see it.

The same two people always paired up. Always finding a reason to be on the same side of the ward. Breaks that somehow line up perfectly, every time.

And you think, right… okay.

Then someone who's been there years will say it casually, like it's nothing:

"Yeah, that's been going on a while."

And that's it. No drama. No big reveal.

Just accepted.

Because it happens everywhere.

Especially in places like this.

There's something about hospital settings in general. The pace, the pressure, the shared experience of dealing with things most people outside don't see.

People talk. Properly talk.

About life, relationships, stress, things they probably wouldn't open up about anywhere else.

And that's where lines can start to blur.

You'll be going about your shift, and suddenly you're aware of things you weren't meant to notice. Conversations that feel a bit too familiar. Glances that last a second longer than they should.

And once you see it, you can't unsee it.

Then comes the unspoken rule:

You mind your business.

Even when it's obvious.

Even when they think they're being subtle—and they're really not.

That's the funny part.

The effort people put into pretending nothing's going on usually makes it more obvious than if they just acted normally.

Different break times. Not sitting near each other. Being overly professional all of a sudden.

It's all part of it.

And over the years, you start to recognise the pattern before it even properly starts.

You'll see two people working together regularly and think:

"Give that a few weeks…"

And more often than not, you're right.

But to be fair, it's not always something to laugh at either.

You realise, as time goes on, that this job can be heavy.

Really heavy.

And people look for connection where they can find it.

Someone who understands the pressure, the pace, the things you see and deal with day in, day out.

It makes sense, in a way.

Even if it's not always the best idea.

Even if it doesn't always end well.

And you do see that side of it, too.

Awkward shifts. People are avoiding each other. That quiet tension when something hasn't worked out the way it was meant to.

But even that becomes part of the background.

People adjust. Things settle. The ward moves on.

It always does.

Looking back over the years, it's just one of those things that sticks out.

Not in a dramatic way.

Just as part of the job.

Part of the environment.

Part of life, really.

You go in thinking you're just there to do your role, look after patients, and get through your shifts.

And you are.

But around all of that, there's a whole other layer—relationships, friendships, connections forming in the middle of everything else.

Some of them last.

Some of them don't.

But they all become part of the story.

And if you've worked long enough in a place like this,

you'll know exactly what I mean—

It happens everywhere.

Part Three, The People Beside You

Chapter 12
The One Who Holds the Line

There's always one.

Not a manager. Not someone with a title that stands out on paper.

Just someone who shows up—consistently, quietly—and somehow makes the shift feel more manageable just by being there.

You don't always notice it at first.

In the beginning, everyone feels the same. Different faces, different personalities, but all part of the same system. You're learning the job, learning the pace, trying to keep up. You don't have time to look too closely at who's who.

But over time, it becomes clear.

There's one person you look for on the rota.

One person who, when you see their name beside yours, you feel something shift—just slightly.

Relief.

Because you know that whatever the shift throws at you, you won't be carrying it alone.

For me, it was them.

No big introductions. No defining moment at the start. Just consistency.

They didn't make a show of things. Didn't try to take control of every situation or prove a point. They just... understood the job. Understood the patients. And, more importantly, understood the people they worked with.

They had a way of reading the room before anything actually happened.

Not reacting, anticipating.

And somehow, they always knew when you needed support, even before you said it out loud.

There was one shift that stayed with me.

Everything about it felt off from the beginning.

One of those days when the ward felt heavier than usual. Patients are more unsettled. Staff stretched thinner than they should have been. Nothing specific you could point to—just a constant underlying tension that sat in the background.

You feel it in your body before anything happens.

That quiet alertness.

Like you're waiting.

I was dealing with a patient who had been escalating throughout the day. Not explosive, not aggressive—just gradually building. Pacing more. Speaking sharper. Less responsive to engagement.

The kind of escalation that can tip either way.

You try everything you're trained to do. De-escalation, conversation, space. Keeping your tone steady, your presence calm.

But you can feel it slipping.

That moment where you realise this might go beyond talking.

And in those seconds, your focus narrows.

You're thinking about the patient, the environment, your own positioning—everything at once. Trying to stay one step ahead without making it obvious.

That's when I noticed them.

Not stepping in. Not taking over.

Just there.

Close enough to support. Far enough to let me work.

Watching everything.

Ready.

It's hard to explain how much that matters in that moment

They didn't say anything straight away.

They didn't need to.

Just knowing they were there changed something.

It steadied you.

Gave you that extra bit of confidence to keep going, to stay present, to not rush or panic.

The situation didn't escalate.

Not fully.

It hovered on that edge for a while, then slowly came back down.

And when it was over—when everything settled, and the ward returned to its usual noise—they didn't make a big deal of it.

No "well done." No breakdown of what happened.

Just a quiet, "You handled that well."

And that was it.

Simple.

But it stayed with me.

Because in a job like this, support isn't always loud.

It's not always stepping in at the last second or taking control.

Sometimes it's just presence.

Knowing someone has your back without needing to say it.

Over time, you start to realise how rare that is.

Not everyone works like that.

Some people bring pressure. Some bring noise. Some make situations harder without meaning to.

But then there are people like them.

The ones who balance things out.

The ones who make you better at your job without even trying to.

The ones who remind you—on the harder days—that you're not doing this alone.

And that matters more than people think.

Because this job can wear you down.

Not just physically.

Mentally.

Emotionally.

In ways that build up over time.

And having even one person who understands that—who notices it, who supports you without making it a thing—can make the difference between getting through a shift and being overwhelmed by it.

I don't think we say it enough.

How much do those people matter?

How much they shape your experience of the job.

How much do they help you stay steady when things feel like they could tip?

You don't always remember every patient.

You don't always remember every shift.

But you remember people like that.

The ones who stood beside you—not in front, not behind—but with you.

Quietly.

Consistently.

Exactly when you needed the support.

Chapter 13
There's Always One

Every hospital has one.

Doesn't matter where you go, how big the place is, how experienced the team is—you'll find them.

The one who is very intelligent.

You can tell straight away.

Well spoken. Confident. Knows all the terminology. Can explain things in a way that sounds impressive—even when you're not entirely sure what they've just said.

And to be fair, they are intelligent.

That's not the issue.

The issue is… when it comes down to the actual job.

It doesn't always translate.

Now, I've come across a few over the years.

Different hospitals, different teams—but somehow, the same pattern.

You'll be on shift, things moving the way they always do—patients needing attention, situations building, decisions needing to be made in real time.

And then you hear it.

"Can I just ask…"

At first, it seems normal.

Of course, you can ask.

We all ask questions.

But then it continues.

"Can I just check…"

"Do you think I should…"

"What would you do if…"

And before you know it, you're being asked about everything.

Every small decision

Every interaction.

Every step.

And you're standing there thinking—

You know this…

Or at least, you should.

It's not that they don't understand things.

They do.

In theory.

But when it comes to actually applying it in the moment, something doesn't quite connect.

And as a manager—or even just someone more experienced—you feel it.

That constant pulling on your attention.

That feeling of being… pestered.

Not in an annoying way at first.

Just constant.

Relentless.

You'll be in the middle of something, and there they are again:

"Sorry, just one more thing…"

And you know it's never just one more thing.

It's five.

Then ten.

And before long, you're answering questions you didn't even know needed answering.

Meanwhile, everything else is still happening around you.

Patients still need you.

The ward still needs you.

And you're trying to balance it all while also being someone else's constant point of reassurance.

That's what it is, really.

Reassurance.

Because underneath all the knowledge, all the confidence on the surface—

There's uncertainty.

And that's not a bad thing.

We've all been there.

But over time, you expect a shift.

A bit more independence.

A bit more trust in their own judgment.

And sometimes… it doesn't come.

They still look to you for everything.

Still double-check things that don't need double-checking.

Still hesitate when a situation calls for action.

And you find yourself wondering how someone so capable on paper can struggle so much in practice.

But then again—that's the thing about this job.

It's not just about knowledge.

It's about instinct.

Presence.

Timing.

Reading people, reading situations, knowing when to step in and when to step back.

And you can't always teach that.

You learn it by being in it.

By getting things wrong sometimes.

By figuring it out as you go.

And not everyone is comfortable with that.

Some people need certainty.

Need to know they're doing it right.

Need someone to confirm it.

And that's where the questions come from.

Constantly.

Over time, you learn how to manage it.

You guide where you can.

Encourage independence.

Give them space to make decisions—even if they're unsure.

Because at some point, they have to trust themselves.

You can't always be there to answer every question

Even if it feels like you already are.

Looking back, it's not something that frustrates me as much as it used to.

If anything, it's just one of those familiar parts of the job.

Because for every one like that—

There's someone else who doesn't ask enough.

Who doesn't check when they should?

And that comes with its own risks.

So maybe it balances out.

But still…

If you've worked in a few different places, you'll know exactly the one I'm talking about.

The one who is clearly intelligent.

Clearly capable.

But somehow still standing beside you, mid-shift, saying:

"Sorry… can I just ask you one more thing?"

All I can say is, I've had to be patient, because they mean well. They really do mean well.

Chapter 14
The Work That Stayed With Me

Looking back, it's not always the crises that stay with me.

It's the quieter work. The kind that doesn't make noise but leaves a mark.

Some of the most memorable projects I was involved in over the years weren't about restraint, or risk, or managing a ward on edge. They were about families.

I remember being part of running family groups, something I didn't think much of at the beginning, if I'm honest. It sounded… structured. Almost too neat for the kind of chaos we were used to dealing with.

But it turned out to be some of the most meaningful work I've ever done.

There's something very different about sitting in a room with families.

Patients, you learn to understand over time. You learn their rhythms, their language, even when it doesn't make sense to anyone else. But families… they come in carrying confusion, fear, frustration, guilt. Sometimes all at once.

And often, no one has really explained things to them in a way that sticks.

I remember one session where we were trying to help families understand how their loved ones might be seeing the world.

Not just clinically. Not just symptoms.

But their reality.

Trying to explain that what looks irrational from the outside can feel completely real to the person experiencing it. That paranoia isn't just suspicion, it's certainty. That voices aren't just thoughts, they're experienced as something external, something present.

You could see it on their faces when it started to click.

Not full understanding, but a shift. A softening.

Less "why are they doing this?"

More "this is what it might feel like for them."

That change matters.

Another part of the group was helping families cope with having a loved one detained under the Mental Health Act.

That word, detained, carries weight.

For families, it can feel like something has been taken out of their hands. Like they've lost control, or even failed in some way. Some felt relief but didn't want to admit it. Others felt anger at the system, at us, sometimes even at their own family member.

And underneath it all, there was often guilt.

We'd sit with that.

Don't fix it. Don't rush it. Just let it be spoken.

Then there were the families struggling with communication.

That quiet frustration of not being able to reach someone you love.

Trying to have a conversation that doesn't land. Asking questions that don't get answers. Or getting responses that don't quite connect.

You could see how exhausting it was for them.

We'd try to help them adjust, not by lowering expectations, but by changing how they approached things. Slowing things down. Giving space. Learning that silence isn't always rejection. That disconnection isn't always intentional.

Short shifts, but important ones.

And then there was the topic that always stirred something in the room, high expressed emotion.

Not everyone liked that term.

It can feel clinical. Judging, even.

But once we unpacked it, the idea that intense criticism, over-involvement, or emotional pressure can actually make things harder for the person who's unwell, it opened up difficult but necessary conversations.

No one wants to hear that the way they show care might be overwhelming the person they love.

But when it was understood properly, it didn't feel like blame.

It felt like insight.

I remember families sitting back, going quiet, reflecting in a way that wasn't defensive, just thoughtful.

Those moments stayed with me.

Because it wasn't about telling people what to do.

It was about helping them see.

And once people see things differently, they often begin to act differently, too.

And then there was something completely different.

An acting group.

I got involved in it almost by chance, staff and patients together, putting something on. I didn't really know what to expect. It could have gone either way, if I'm honest.

But it worked.

It really worked.

We'd come together, rehearse, and laugh more than anything else. There was something about it that stripped everything back. No labels. No "staff" and "patient" in the usual sense.

Just people.

People are trying to remember lines, getting them wrong, starting again. People stepping into roles that weren't defined by illness or profession.

And you'd see sides of people you wouldn't normally see on the ward.

Confidence where there hadn't been any.

Humour that doesn't always come out in clinical conversations.

Connection that just… happened.

We put on a small play in the end.

Nothing huge. Nothing polished in a professional sense.

But that wasn't the point.

We performed it during an open day, families there, staff around, a different kind of atmosphere to the usual ward environment.

And it was brilliant.

It really was.

There was something powerful about watching patients stand up and perform, not as "patients", but as themselves, or even as someone else entirely. For that moment, they weren't defined by why they were in hospital.

They were just part of something.

So were we.

I remember enjoying it more than I expected to. Actually looking forward to it.

It felt light, and that's not something you get to say often in this job.

No pressure. No edge. Just a shared effort to create something, however small.

Looking back, those moments matter just as much as the heavier ones.

Maybe more.

Because they remind you that there's more to people than their worst days.

And sometimes, if you give the space for it…

That part shows up.

Part Four, The Other Shift, and Why I Stayed

Chapter 15
The Other Shift, Motherhood

People often talk about how hard nursing is.

The long hours.

The emotional toll.

The responsibility.

And it is all of those things.

But what people don't always see… is what happens when your shift doesn't end when you leave the hospital.

Because for some of us, there's another shift waiting at home.

Motherhood.

Working full-time as a nurse and having two young children… I don't even know where to begin with that.

It's not just busy.

It's constant.

Your day doesn't start when you clock in; it starts early in the morning, before your shift, when you're getting little ones ready. Trying to get yourself sorted while making breakfast, packing bags, finding missing shoes, calming tears over something that feels big to them but small to you… But it still matters.

You're already "on duty" before you even leave the house.

Then you go to work.

And work is work.

You don't get to say, "I'm tired today, I've had a long morning." Patients still need you. The ward is still busy. People still rely on you to be switched on, present, calm, especially in mental health, where how you show up matters just as much as what you do.

So you push through.

You give your all, because that's what we do.

And then the shift ends.

But it doesn't really end.

You go home… and it starts again.

"Ma'am!"

"Mom!"

"I'm hungry."

"Can you help me?"

"Watch this!"

And in that moment, no matter how tired you are, you switch roles instantly.

Because to them, you're not a nurse.

You're everything.

There were days I came home absolutely exhausted. Physically drained. Mentally full from everything I had seen, heard, and held throughout the day.

And still…

Dinner had to be made.

Baths had to be done.

Stories had to be read.

There's no pause button.

I remember thinking sometimes, how am I doing this?

How are any of us doing this?

Because there's no real break.

Even on your days off, you're still "on".

School runs. Activities. Appointments. Trying to be present, trying not to let the exhaustion take over.

And then the guilt creeps in.

The guilt of being at work and not being with your children.

The guilt of being with your children but feeling too tired to give them 100%.

It's a constant push-and-pull.

You're torn between two worlds that both need you fully.

And you try.

You really do try.

I remember nights where I'd sit down after putting the kids to bed, and that would be the first moment I'd had to myself all day.

And sometimes I'd just sit there in silence.

Too tired to even move.

Too tired to even think.

But then… Some moments make it all worth it.

The hugs when you walk through the door.

The "I missed you."

The little stories they tell you about their day, like it's the most important thing in the world.

And it is.

Because they don't see the tiredness.

They don't see the stress.

They just see you.

And somehow, that gives you a second wind.

Working as a nurse teaches you resilience.

But motherhood?

That teaches you a different kind of strength.

A quieter one.

A deeper one.

The kind where you keep going, not because you have to, but because people you love depend on you.

Looking back, I don't think I gave myself enough credit.

I was just doing what needed to be done.

Like so many others.

But now I realise…

Juggling both isn't just "managing".

It's surviving.

It's adapting.

It's loving two roles at once, even when they pull you in different directions.

And to anyone doing both, working in healthcare and raising children —

I see you.

Because it's not easy.

But somehow… we do it.

Every single day.

Chapter 16
The Life You Miss While Living It

Social life.

I suppose this also ties into work-life balance, or, if I'm being honest, the lack of it.

Having a social life as a nurse isn't as simple as people think.

It's actually very difficult.

You don't really have one unless you make one for yourself. And even then, it takes planning, effort, and sometimes a bit of luck.

We work long hours.

12-hour shifts. Sometimes longer.

By the time you finish, you're not thinking about going out or meeting friends, you're thinking about getting home, having something to eat, and going straight to bed.

You're physically tired.

But more than that, you're mentally drained.

Especially in mental health.

You've spent the whole day talking, listening, observing, managing emotions, other people's emotions, and holding things that don't just disappear when your shift ends.

So when you finally leave work, sometimes the last thing you want to do is be around more people.

You just want quiet.

You want space.

You want to switch off.

And then there's your friends.

A lot of my friends are nurses too.

Which sounds ideal, because they understand the job. They get the stress, the long hours, the emotional side of things.

But in reality, it makes things harder.

Because you're all working different shifts.

Opposite shifts.

Somebody's on an early. Someone else is on a late. Someone is on nights. Someone is off but recovering from nights.

So you don't see each other.

Not properly.

You have to plan everything.

And when I say plan, I mean really plan.

Dinners are booked months in advance. Sometimes six months. Sometimes even a year.

You look forward to it.

You finally think, "Right, we're going to meet. We're going to catch up."

And then…

"Sorry, I can't make it."

"My shift got changed."

"They cancelled my leave."

"I've been asked to cover."

And just like that, it's off.

Again.

It happens so often that after a while, you almost expect it.

You don't even get disappointed the same way anymore.

You just say, "Yeah, no worries," and carry on.

But deep down… it does affect you.

Because over time, you realise how much you've missed.

Birthdays.

Dinners.

Simple catch-ups.

Moments that other people take for granted.

And it's not just friendships.

I've seen marriages struggle.

I've seen relationships fall apart.

Not because people didn't love each other, but because they didn't have the time.

Different shifts.

Opposite schedules.

Constant tiredness.

You miss each other without even realising it.

You're passing like ships.

One coming in, one going out.

And over time, that distance builds.

That's the reality people don't always talk about.

This job doesn't just affect you, it affects your relationships too.

I think that's something I didn't fully acknowledge at the time.

I was just getting on with things.

Working. Living. Managing.

But when I look back now, I can see it more clearly.

I missed out on a lot socially.

Before, I used to really try.

I'd make the effort. I'd push myself to go out, even when I was tired.

But now… I find it harder.

Maybe it's because I've moved.

Maybe it's just life.

Most of my close friends now live in different parts of the world.

And even the ones I do have around me, they have their own lives, their own families, their own responsibilities.

And again, different schedules.

Different shifts.

So it becomes even harder to line things up.

And that's where it can get a bit lonely.

Not in a dramatic way.

But in a quiet, subtle way.

The kind where you realise you haven't seen a friend in months.

The kind where your conversations happen more over messages than in person.

The kind where you say, "We must meet soon," and you both mean it… But it just doesn't happen.

And people don't really talk about that side of the job.

The impact it has on your social life.

The impact it has on relationships.

The mental toll it can take.

Because as human beings, we need connection.

We need friendships.

We need our partners.

We need laughter, conversations, and being around people who know us outside of work.

We need to be something other than "the nurse".

But when you're constantly working, constantly tired, constantly trying to catch up on life, it becomes difficult.

Even on your days off, you're not always available.

You're recovering.

Catching up on sleep.

Doing house chores.

Sorting out everything you didn't have time to do during your working days.

Food shopping. Cleaning. Life admin.

And before you know it, your days off are gone.

And you still haven't seen anyone.

Even the idea of going out can feel like an effort.

Because you've already given so much of yourself.

Physically. Mentally. Emotionally.

And sometimes, you just don't have anything left to give.

I think that's something people don't always understand.

A lot of people work 9 to 5.

They have evenings free. Weekends off. A routine.

We don't.

Our lives are unpredictable.

Our schedules change.

And that comes at a cost.

A social cost.

An emotional cost.

But if there's one thing I've learned, and I'm still learning it —

It's that you have to be intentional.

You have to make time.

Because it won't just happen.

You have to create it.

Not just for friends, but for your family, for your partner, for the people who matter most.

Even if it's small.

Even if it's just a coffee instead of a big night out.

Even if it's just sitting down together without distractions.

Even if you're tired.

Make time.

Because relationships need time.

They need presence.

They need effort.

Make time for your friends.

Make time for your family.

Make time for your partner.

Make time for yourself.

Because it matters.

It really does.

It's not just about socialising.

It's about connection.

It's about balance.

It's about protecting the parts of your life that exist outside of work.

Because this job, as much as we love it, can take over if we let it.

So to anyone reading this, not just nurses, but anyone —

Don't wait for the "right time".

Make the time.

Call that friend.

Send that message.

Sit with your partner.

Plan that dinner, even if it gets cancelled three times before it actually happens.

And sometimes…

Just go out.

Just laugh.

Just be.

Because you need it.

And you deserve it.

Chapter 17
It Takes a Village

I can't not add a little about my support system

They say it takes a village.

And to be fair—coming from where I come from—I believe that.

Because if I really started listing everyone who's supported me over the years, the book would be a million pages long. Family, friends, people who stepped in at the right time, people who showed up when I didn't even realise I needed them.

It really does take a whole village.

But if I'm being honest, there are a few who carry more than their fair share.

And for me, that's my children.

Now, I don't know how it happened, but somewhere along the way, I ended up with two people who seem to understand me better than I understand myself half the time.

My daughter and my son.

Amazing kids.

And I'm not just saying that because I'm their parent.

They've seen me through all versions of myself. The tired version, the stressed version, the "don't talk to me, I've just come off a long shift" version.

And somehow… they still like me.

Which, considering everything, is impressive.

There's something about coming home after a long day—one of those shifts where everything has taken a bit out of you—and just being able to sit, exist, and not have to explain yourself.

They get it.

I don't always have to say, "Today was hard."

They can see it.

And instead of asking a hundred questions, they just… adjust.

Give you space when you need it.

Or distract you when they know that's what you need more.

Sometimes it's the smallest things.

A random conversation about something completely unrelated to work.

A bit of laughter when you didn't even realise you needed it.

Or just their presence—normal, steady, grounding.

And it reminds you that there's a whole world outside of the hospital.

Because it's very easy to get pulled into that world completely.

To let it take over more space than it should.

But they pull you back without even trying.

Keep you balanced.

Keep you human.

And then—just when you think life couldn't get any fuller—

along come the grandbabies.

Now, no one prepares you for that level of joy.

Or that level of energy, to be honest.

You think you've done your time raising kids, you've earned a bit of peace… and then suddenly you're back to chasing little humans around again.

But this time, it's different.

Because you get all the good parts.

The laughter, the cuddles, the chaos—and then, when they've completely worn you out…

You can hand them back.

Which, I won't lie, is one of the best parts.

But jokes aside, they bring something into your life that you can't really explain.

A kind of lightness.

A reminder not to take everything so seriously.

Because no matter how heavy work gets, no matter how much you carry from one shift to the next—

They don't see any of that.

To them, you're just you.

And that does something.

It resets you.

Reminds you who you are outside the uniform, outside the responsibility, outside everything that comes with the job.

Looking back, I can honestly say I wouldn't have managed this career the way I have without them.

Without that support.

Without that constant presence in the background, holding everything steady.

So yes, it takes a village.

And I'm grateful for all of mine.

But if I'm being real—

my children…

and my grandbabies…

They're the ones who keep me going

more than they'll probably ever realise.

Chapter 18
Why I Stayed

I've often wondered how to end this.

Not just the book... but the job itself.

Because nursing doesn't really have a clean ending.

There's no final shift where everything is tied together. No moment where you sit back and say, " That's it, that's everything wrapped up neatly.

It doesn't work like that.

Even now, after all these years, I still walk out of shifts carrying pieces with me.

Some days it's light.

Other days... not so much.

Faces stay with you.

Not all of them. But some.

The ones who said something small that stuck.

The ones who didn't say anything at all.

The ones you worried about, even after handing over.

You don't always know what happens to people when they leave your care.

Sometimes you see them again. Sometimes you don't.

And that's one of the hardest parts, learning to be part of someone's life, even if only for a moment, and then letting go.

No closure.

No full story.

Just a piece.

I've seen a lot over the years.

Good days.

Bad days.

Days that felt like they would never end.

I've seen people at their lowest, and I've seen them come back from it.

I've seen strength in places you wouldn't expect.

And vulnerability in people who looked like they had everything together.

I've seen colleagues hold things together when they were falling apart themselves.

And I've seen how this job can take from you, slowly, over time.

Your energy.

Your patience.

Sometimes, even parts of who you were before you started.

But it also gives you something.

Not in a loud, obvious way.

In a quieter way.

It teaches you how to sit with people in their worst moments, without needing to fix everything.

It teaches you that not all progress is visible.

That sometimes just being there is enough.

It teaches you to listen… properly listen.

Not to respond. Not to correct.

Just to understand.

And maybe the biggest thing it teaches you is this:

People are more than their worst day.

That applies to patients.

And if I'm honest… it applies to us too.

Because there were days I didn't get it right.

Days I was tired, distracted, stretched too thin.

Days I walked away thinking, I could have done better.

But you don't get to go back.

You just come in the next day and try again.

That's the job.

Not perfection.

Just showing up. Again and again.

I've written about a lot, the pressure, the loneliness, the difficult moments, the things people don't always see.

And all of that is real.

But so is this:

There were moments of connection.

Moments of understanding.

Moments where something small shifted, and you knew it mattered.

Even if no one else saw it.

Even if it wasn't written in any notes.

Just a look.

A conversation.

A quiet "thank you."

Those moments stay with you, too.

Maybe more than anything else.

If there's one thing I've learned, it's that this job isn't about having all the answers.

It's about being there, even when there aren't any.

Standing in the middle of uncertainty and still choosing to care.

Even when you're tired.

Even when the system is stretched.

Even when it would be easier to switch off.

You still show up.

And that's something.

I don't know how long I'll keep doing this.
I don't think many of us do.
But for now… I'm still here.
Still walking onto the ward.
Still doing the job.
And at the end of the day…
You take a breath,
step outside,
and leave what you can behind.
And somehow…
You come back again.

www.ingramcontent.com/pod-product-compliance
Lightning Source LLC
LaVergne TN
LVHW100732061126
851857LV00011B/501
9781066632640